"Based on his Christian convictions and years of treating the marginalized, Dr. Cutillo calls for reorienting the philosophy and practice of medicine. A society consumed by a delusional drive for invulnerability needs to look to the truths of creation and the fall and of the incarnation and resurrection of Jesus: humans are finite and mortal, yet there is hope in the fact that God took on flesh and conquered death. Eloquently argued with references to philosophy, literature, and theology, this volume urges readers to redefine the relationship between faith and medicine. A profound, timely book."

M. Daniel Carroll R., Professor of Old Testament, Wheaton College Graduate School; author, *Christians at the Border*

"Dr. Cutillo challenges his medical colleagues and the Christian church to look at how health care is provided in the context of modern medicine and in light of what the Bible teaches about caring for one another in today's global society. His heart for and experience in caring for the poor and underserved along with his study of the Bible inform this excellent presentation of the issues as they have evolved historically."

Grace J. Tazellar, Missions Director, Nurses Christian Fellowship; author, *Caring Across Cultures*

"Few people could have written this book with the penetrating perspective of Dr. Cutillo. He has a unique viewpoint from medical practice in some of the best Christian health centers in the US and abroad that helps him to understand health care. His medical perspective leads him to an eloquent but gentle lament for medicine's impersonal 'disembodiment,' as it divides patients into organ systems, statistics, and computerized templates. However, his theological training and wide reading of the classics help us clearly see ways in which the integration of faith into health care can make it more truly caring. Dr. Cutillo's conclusion draws on the hope he has learned from suffering patients and the joy he has witnessed as the result of true Christian community. He offers a positive change of direction I find very compelling. Read and be inspired."

John Payne, MD, President, Medical Ambassadors International; Former Family Medicine Residency Director, University of California, Davis

"Health care has begun to feel like a zero-sum game. Struggles over coverages and copays have often supplanted thoughts about health itself. Our focus on the technologies, institutions, and politics of health care delivery have superseded considerations (and conversations) about the integration of health with biblical faith, community, and justice. Into this fraught space, Dr. Cutillo has introduced an astute thoughtfulness that is challenging, refreshing, and deeply grounded. His incisive analysis is delivered in a way that is ˑˑ ˑ inviting. This doctor has great bedside manner!"

David M. Erickson, President and CI

D1468363

"This excellent resource, beginning with the simple conviction that health is a gift given by God, will challenge the way you and our culture look at medicine and health care. Whether Dr. Cutillo is discussing the proper care for our bodies, the proper place of science in health care, how we face death, or how to properly steward precious health care resources for the good of all, this book will inform and challenge some of your most basic, and perhaps incorrect, assumptions about medicine and health care."

Walt Larimore, MD, best-selling author, *10 Essentials of Happy, Healthy People* and *Workplace Grace: Becoming a Spiritual Influence at Work*

"Cutillo's vision of how faith and medicine can cooperate offers an anecdote to the anxiety that diminishes personal health and contributes to defensive medicine. Of particular interest is Cutillo's treatment of how anxiety and fear lead to self-absorption, consequently contributing to health disparities and injustice. With the church having the antidote to anxiety in the gospel, what might happen to the health of our communities if we lived fully into that message? A must read for those who are concerned about integrating faith and health in their professional practice or ministry."

Mary Chase-Ziolek, Professor of Health Ministries and Nursing, North Park University and Seminary; author, *Health, Healing, and Wholeness*

"Bob Cutillo is an amazing doctor with vast experience in delivering health care in several contexts. He is extremely well qualified to guide us in our understanding of health care in the anxious days ahead. Dr. Cutillo uses his expertise and experience to help us think through health care with a hopeful mind-set. I highly recommend *Pursuing Health in an Anxious Age*."

Wayne "Coach" Gordon, Pastor, Lawndale Christian Community Church, Chicago

"Reflection on the moral meaning of medicine sometimes results in contrived collections of guidelines or flowcharts to assist in making difficult medical decisions. In a refreshing alternative, Dr. Cutillo has woven a wise and engaging meditation with the power to transform how we imagine the meaning of health and of community. By situating the practice of medicine in the context of modernity's preoccupations, obsessions, and blind spots, he reminds us that health is neither an entitlement nor a reductionist solution to an engineering problem. It is, rather, a gift—given by one who took on human form himself—to be received and cherished with wonder and love."

Ken Myers, host and producer, *Mars Hill Audio Journal*

Pursuing Health in an Anxious Age

Pursuing Health in an Anxious Age

Bob Cutillo, MD

Foreword by Andy Crouch

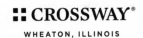

WHEATON, ILLINOIS

Pursuing Health in an Anxious Age

Copyright © 2016 by Bob Cutillo, MD

Published by Crossway
        1300 Crescent Street
        Wheaton, Illinois 60187

Cover design: Tim Green, Faceout Studio

Cover image: © AGorohov / Shutterstock

First printing 2016

Printed in the United States of America

Unless otherwise indicated, Scripture quotations are taken from The Holy Bible, New International Version®, NIV®. Copyright © 1973, 1978, 1984, 2011 by Biblica, Inc.™ Used by permission. All rights reserved worldwide.

Scripture references marked NRSV are from *The New Revised Standard Version*. Copyright © 1989 by the Division of Christian Education of the National Council of the Churches of Christ in the U.S.A. Published by Thomas Nelson, Inc. Used by permission of the National Council of the Churches of Christ in the U.S.A.

All emphases in Scripture quotations have been added by the author.

Trade paperback ISBN: 978-1-4335-5110-9
ePub ISBN: 978-1-4335-5113-0
PDF ISBN: 978-1-4335-5111-6
Mobipocket ISBN: 978-1-4335-5112-3

Library of Congress Cataloging-in-Publication Data

Names: Cutillo, Bob, 1955- author.

Title: Pursuing health in an anxious age / Bob Cutillo, MD ; foreword by Andy Crouch.

Description: Wheaton : Crossway, 2016. | Series: The Gospel coalition (faith and work) | Includes bibliographical references and index.

Identifiers: LCCN 2016012083 (print) | LCCN 2016022137 (ebook) | ISBN 9781433551109 (tp) | ISBN 9781433551130 (epub) | ISBN 9781433551116 (pdf) | ISBN 9781433551123 (mobi)

Subjects: LCSH: Health—Religious aspects—Christianity.

Classification: LCC BT732 .C88 2016 (print) | LCC BT732 (ebook) | DDC 248.4—dc23

LC record available at https://lccn.loc.gov/2016012083

Crossway is a publishing ministry of Good News Publishers.

VP   26 25 24 23 22 21 20 19 18 17 16
15 14 13 12 11 10 9 8 7 6 5 4 3 2 1

To my mother, Francine

Contents

Foreword

Perhaps once a year, if I am lucky, I encounter a book that addresses a supremely important topic and does so in a supremely helpful way. This is such a book, and I am thrilled to be introducing it here.

What are we to do with our bodies, fearfully and wonderfully made as they are, in times of illness, vulnerability, and death? That question has always been with us. But it is becoming especially urgent for the citizens of the technological world—or, more baldly put, subjects of the technological empire that holds out to us a vision of the good life buttressed by scientific knowledge but also demands from us ever more loyalty and obedience.

As a citizen of that empire, it feels almost subversive to observe that there is something uniquely tragic about our age of modern medicine—tragic in the old sense of genuine greatness and good intentions turned awry by a fatal flaw.

In so many ways, medicine has delivered real cures and relief of suffering. It's likely that I am here to write this foreword, forty-eight years into my mortal life, only because of the direct and indirect contributions of medicine, starting with the vaccines that warded off many a childhood illness, the antibiotics that effortlessly cured many another, the anesthesia that has made minor but essential surgeries possible, and the more mundane benefits of dentistry and ophthalmology, just to name a few. And for the most part, the human beings who have prescribed and delivered these treatments have been people of intelligence, wisdom, patience, and kindness—bearers of the *imago Dei* at their best.

Yet in so many other ways, medicine falls ever short of our

expectations that it will deliver us from the basic human condition, the morbidity and mortality that are our inheritance as fallen creatures. There is an abiding tension between medicine's achievements, which are tremendous; its promises, which at the limit are nothing less than "You shall be like God" and, above all, "You shall not surely die"; and its strangely persistent failure to bring the real flourishing that we long for, either for practitioners or for patients.

The increasingly crushing demands on many medical professionals, the dwindling time available for real encounter and empathy between physicians and patients, the costs that escalate year after year beyond many families' (and perhaps, ultimately, our whole society's) ability to afford, the heroic but expensive attempts to stave off the end of life that often lead to persons spending their final days enmeshed in a brutalist matrix of life-support machines—all of this seems to suggest that something has gone wrong in the story of medical progress. And on the horizon are potentially catastrophic developments, including the possibility that our time will be remembered as the single brief moment when antibiotics actually were effective, before the rise of invulnerable bacteria that escaped from the hospitals (where they are already alarmingly entrenched) into the wider world.

Then there is the question of what lengths we will go to, as our expectations from medicine continue to escalate, to keep the stream of medical breakthroughs coming. What if it turns out that creating, exploiting, and destroying human lives can provide us the raw material—from stem cells to entire organs—to cure the diseases, or even just satisfy the desires for enhancement, of the wealthy and powerful? Why and how will we resist that new and more sophisticated form of child sacrifice?

We will only realize the real promise of medicine, it seems to me, and resist its transformation into the most horrifying of idolatries, if we discover a new vision for being human, one that values vulnerability as much as control, community as much as autonomy, and mystery as much as certainty.

That is the way that Dr. Bob Cutillo offers in this book, and one of the many great gifts of this book is that rather than simply critiquing our current medical culture (as I fear I've done in these paragraphs), he offers a positively beautiful account of how a human-scale practice of medicine can actually fulfill our deepest desires in ways that merely technological medicine, for all its grandiose promises, can never achieve. This is a vision of health that is far richer than mere test results or statistics—it is embedded in community, informed by story and literature, and ultimately rooted in prayer and praise.

It is crucial that Dr. Cutillo's own story, and the perspective of this book, includes providing care to the most vulnerable, especially those who live in neglected neighborhoods in our own country. By constantly reframing his assessment of medicine through the experience of people whose lives do not fit any neat picture of affluent flourishing, he recalls all of us to a picture of health that goes deeper than you'll find in carefully crafted pharmaceutical advertisements or expensive downtown gyms. By telling their stories of life and death, illness and health, with sympathetic attention, he invites us to pay deeper attention to our own stories, slowing down our frenzied pursuit of relief from every small distress.

What we see in these pages is the beginning of a better way for all of us, a kind of health that we've almost forgotten is possible. One of my favorite phrases in the whole Bible comes when Paul is instructing his younger partner Timothy in how to pastor the wealthy in his congregation. He urges Timothy to lead them toward "the life that really is life" (1 Tim. 6:19 NRSV). If there is a life that really is life, there must also be a health that really is health. If we read and heed this book, we may still be able to find it.

Andy Crouch,
author; executive editor, *Christianity Today*

Preface

It was during my years as a medical student in New York City that I first began to wonder: Why do we fragment a patient into pieces to give good medical care? And why do we segregate the rich and insured from the poor and uninsured to deliver good health care?

One night during the first year, worn out by the overwhelming number of facts I was learning in books about the human body, I took a walk to the hospital, where I met a young man from Harlem. He was in the medical ward, a large room with fifteen to twenty beds, where the only privacy available was a curtain pulled around the bed. (Not surprisingly, the rich and famous of New York were in another part of the hospital.) He was there in a sickle-cell crisis, and I was there in a personal one. Though I was too early in training to offer anything of medical value, I offered my interest in him and a desire to sit and talk. Listening to his story that night and hearing of the things that had hindered his health and the way he had been treated in the health care system, I knew I needed a bigger view.

The years since have only confirmed these suspicions. I see it on the faces of patients who fear that the institution of medicine and those who work within it will forget them as persons while treating them as patients. I feel it in the loss of many good colleagues who leave the practice of medicine too young and too soon, still with so much care to give but too tired to focus on patients while trying to follow the rules and regulations of a complex and unjust health care system. And I know it in the failure of our culture to offer a reasonable view of who we are as human beings and how we fit in the communities we inhabit.

Instead of accepting the thinking that medicine and religion should remain apart, perhaps it is only a theological turn that can save us. But a theological investigation can never be a simple application of ready-made, clear-cut answers to human questions. If applied science demands direct results, applied theology first asks for a change in vision. In wrestling with a particular darkness but always moving toward a particular light, a new vision will change what we are doing, but only after clarifying where we are going.

As a practitioner of medicine and a student of the cultural context in which we pursue health, this venture in applied theology depends on two points of reference. The first vantage point is that of orthodox Christian belief. Thus it is toward the light of Christ that this work looks, using that light to explore how we pursue health and practice health care. Some will by upbringing or personal faith be attracted to this perspective; others may find it a strange and unlikely place from which to look.

The other vantage point is from the margins, with the medically disenfranchised, where I have been for most of my career. In trying to bring the least, the lost, and the left out into our models of care, I have found many barriers but also a great deal of health and healing just by being in their midst. Some who find the former stance comfortable may be uneasy with some of the conclusions drawn here. Yet those who start from an uneasy view of theology may find much with which they resonate in this latter perspective.

Whatever the case may be, for those who desire to see a deeper response to the care of the sick and the protection of the healthy in an anxious age, I invite you into this exploration. We will always be limited to the vision given by the particular vantage points from which we look. This book reflects my love of medicine and my belief in the church. My highest hope is that I have been faithful to what I have seen and heard from the places where I have stood.

A book of this nature, with hard questions concerning big issues, cannot come into being without many arms outstretched to lift up, to hold back, or to point the way. In the beginning there was Bethany Jenkins at The Gospel Coalition, who first saw that this book was important, that it was possible, and that someone like me could write it. Others may have thought so sooner, but she was the first one who knew what lay ahead yet still believed despite the obstacles. Her comments throughout the preparation of the manuscript helped to sharpen and balance it on numerous occasions.

I am indebted beyond measure to the thoughts of others, particularly those who wrote before me, many far back and, often in accord with the distance, with penetrating prophecy. The printed word, as Edmund Fuller says, "gives us extraordinary freedom to choose the intellectual company we will keep, to select those with whom, in spirit, we will walk. It is a privilege . . . in the highest sense it is a duty. . . . Paraphrasing Joshua, 'Choose this day whom you will read.'"[1] I was fortunate to choose wisely on many occasions.

Several of the authors whose words became windows through which to make sense of my world I met through the excellent work of *Mars Hill Audio Journal*. With host Ken Myers's interviews carefully revealing his guests' best ideas, it often led me on a fruitful journey of further reading. I am indebted to Gary VanderPol for introducing me to the work of Charles Taylor and also thank him for his thoughtful feedback on the early stages of this book.

Writing is also soul searching, with unknown passages and caves where bottoms suddenly drop out, and you don't know where you are. That can be frightening. I thank Cindy, Dave, Gary, Jennifer, Mark, Pam, and Steve, whose promise of prayer often strengthened me, smoothing out many a bump and pushing me forward when I wasn't sure where I was going or whether I could get there.

The skilled and gifted team at Crossway have performed a remarkable service in directing me through the labyrinth of publication. They suggested and directed, and, like the push and pull of sandpaper across rough wood, smoothed and polished the writing into better form. But above all and before any of this, it was their courage to risk I most admire, when they first entertained the idea of publishing this book.

I have been warmed at the hearth and fired in the furnace of several health care homes. I am indeed grateful for the formation I received at Lawndale Christian Health Center in Chicago; Kintambo Centre de Santé in Kinshasa; Christ House and Columbia Road Health Services in Washington, DC; and Inner City Health Center and Colorado Coalition for the Homeless Stout Street Health Center in Denver.

My deepest gratitude is for my wife, Heather. Because of her constant companionship over the last thirty years of the journey, only she knew what I was trying to say even before I could say it. Over countless conversations at breakfasts and much longer walks in the parks and mountains of Colorado, she kept reminding me what I meant to say, and as the first reader of everything I wrote, she gave me constant hope that I could do it. If richness is in relationships, no one can exceed the wealth I have in my wife.

I thank my children, Kate and Steve, and their spouses, Tim and Rachel, for their love, their support, and their ongoing commitment to live life honestly and faithfully in a challenging age.

Finally, I stand in awe of the courage and candor of numerous patients over many years. Though I would like to say that everyone taught me something, it is more honest to admit that I wasn't always listening. But I never stopped believing that what the next patient might say or do was important, and so much of what was offered I was able to receive. Seeing life through their eyes—the eyes of those in fear and hope, in love, in pain and suffering, and in passive resignation or righteous indignation that no one cared about those like them at the margins—was a gift of great value. It was they who opened the window through which I could see my own culture in sober view.

Introduction

What Is Health For?

The greatest wealth is health.

Virgil

Health has always been cherished but never controlled. In 19 BC, Virgil, one of Rome's greatest poets, went to Greece to work on revisions of his most famous poem, the *Aeneid*. On his way back home, he caught a fever, arrived in Italy weakened by disease, and died in harbor. Though he was only fifty years old, he had already lived longer than expected for his time.[1] With little to do when sickness arrived, his awareness of the value of health only emphasized how fragile and precious life is.

American poet and essayist Ralph Waldo Emerson also believed, "The first wealth is health." When he died in 1882, life expectancy was still less than fifty years. He, too, did not expect a great deal of control over health, living before the discovery of painless surgery under anesthesia, or the knowledge of a microbial world whose infections could be prevented with hygiene or treated with antibiotics.

Things have changed a great deal since then. We now live in a world with greater health and more health care than ever before. Life expectancy in most industrialized countries nears eighty years of age.

Diseases such as tuberculosis, which caused the death of Emerson's wife at age nineteen, can now be cured. Never before has the horizon for health looked so bright or the choices for health care been so varied. From organ transplants to respirators to cancer treatments to genetic mapping, the future seems unlimited, each boundary but a temporary pause in the march of progress.

Yet higher levels of health and greater quantities of health care, rather than creating greater peace and prosperity for all, have been associated with some troubling side effects—greater worry, increased waste, and a waylaid commitment to care for the health of our neighbor.

More Control but Greater Worry

When Joyce and her husband, Samuel, discovered they were pregnant for the first time, she was a graduate student in philosophy. Having delayed starting a family for several years while they pursued further education, getting pregnant at an older age was not as easy as they had planned. But over a year of waiting only made the positive pregnancy test that much more exciting.

They shared their joy with family and friends. Joyce's sister, a mother of three, told them how important it was to start getting checkups right away and recommended that they see her midwife. But Samuel's brother, Jacob, a doctor, was concerned that she was high risk because of her older age and recommended a friend of his who was an obstetrician. As usual when the family was dealing with medical issues, Jacob's advice could not be refused, and on a Tuesday morning one week later they went to see Dr. Abernathy.

He entered the room with apologies for being late. Despite feeling rushed by a full schedule of patients, he took time to review the forms Joyce had filled out, asked one or two questions for clarification, and performed a careful exam and ultrasound. Afterward, he returned to the room to discuss next steps. "Joyce, the ultrasound confirms the date of your pregnancy at two months. Though I see nothing abnormal at this point, I recommend doing further testing to see if the baby is healthy. After all, you've waited so long. There are always risks of abnormalities, but at your age it is more likely. Down syndrome is the most common, but there are other problems that are much more severe, even incompatible with life. You do want to take advantage of all the options to insure the health of your baby, don't you?"

Later that day, as Joyce and Samuel thought back on their visit, three things stood out. First, though Dr. Abernathy was harried, he was genuinely interested in providing high-quality care. Second, they remembered how efficient everyone was, particularly the nurse who came in later to answer their questions about the recommended testing. Finally, and most significantly, they realized something had changed. Tuesday morning they had gone to the office happy and excited, wondering if they would find out whether they were having a boy or a girl. Tuesday night they were worried and afraid. Was their baby physically deformed or mentally defective? Had they waited too long to get pregnant? What tests should they do? What would they do if they found something wrong?

What happened to Joyce and Samuel is not unusual in today's health care encounter. On several occasions I have met parents-to-be just like them. The joy of discovering they are pregnant can be one of the purest in life. But upon entering the medical system, their wonder and awe at a gift received shrivel before efforts to calculate unknown risks, worries about what bad things could happen, and fretful decisions about how to manage the pregnancy to obtain a quality outcome. How quickly the power to control an unpredictable future and the great possibilities to maximize health can transform joy and hope into calculation and concern. Whether in preparation for childbirth, making preventive health choices, or considering treatment options for cancer or end-of-life decisions, worry has become one of the marks of modern health care.

More Health Care but Increased Waste

Not surprisingly, more health care costs more money. From 1960 to 2010 the percentage of the Gross Domestic Product (GDP) spent on health care in the United States more than tripled, to nearly 18 percent. At about 2.8 trillion dollars, it was more than four times the amount dedicated to defense and three times the amount for education.[2] On top of that, individual consumers spend an additional one hundred billion dollars on fitness programs, anti-aging procedures, dietary programs and supplements, and cosmetic skin care products.[3] Are we spending too much for health care? If health is our greatest wealth, can it ever be too much? That's hard to say—unless what we spend is wasteful.

The best estimates are that up to 30 percent of the money we spend on health care is of little or no value.[4] Many factors contribute to this problem. Much of health care is fragmented—tests are often repeated and unnecessary medicines prescribed because one health care provider does not know what the other is doing. Unfair pricing produces costs that have little to do with value—patients are often shocked to look at an itemized hospital bill and find a gauze pad costing ten dollars. Doctors practice defensive medicine for fear of being sued, provide treatments to fulfill standard protocols irrespective of particular situations, or order tests rather than talk to patients, because they have so little time. The list goes on, but the result is the same—we end up paying for health care that conveys little or no benefit. And if that weren't enough cause for concern, what if wasteful spending and too much health care for some means too little for others?

More for Some, Less for Others

The third disturbing trend is our waylaid commitment to caring for our neighbor. As some of us worry about what we can do to insure our personal health and spend larger amounts on things that have little or no benefit, others struggle for even the most basic services. Over the last thirty years, in conjunction with the rapid growth in health care spending and services, the number of uninsured in the United States has steadily climbed.[5] The uninsured have greater difficulty finding access to health care than those with insurance, causing neglect of health problems, sickness at more advanced stages, and higher death rates.[6] This seems unwise and unjust in a country that spends as much money on health care as the United States does.

Yet the plight of the uninsured in this country, or the poor and marginalized in general, is easily lost in the heated debates over health care reform. In 2012 we spent more than twice per person on health care than most economically developed countries, including France,

Germany, or Japan,[7] and more than five hundred times what is spent for a person living in economically depressed countries such as the Democratic Republic of Congo.[8] Yet the gap continues to grow as fear of losing control of our personal health strains the fabric of concern for the common good. With tunnel-vision focus on how changes in the financing and delivery of health care will affect *my* health care, we have little room for our neighbor at home and even greater neglect of the huge disparities in global health for our neighbors far away.

The Many Faces of Health Care

As we struggle to understand the worry, waste, and waylaid commitment to others in an age with more stability, certainty, and safety in health than ever before, it may be helpful to consider how complicated health care has become as our expectations for it have grown. No longer just a doctor-patient relationship, it is a complex system with many faces. Spend one day in a hospital bed and you will see it from many angles.

In the morning your doctor visits you. Her careful attention to the facts of medicine gives you confidence that you are receiving the best tests and treatment. If health care is to be dependably good, it must be scientifically sound. *Health care requires good science.*

But today the science is not certain. Yesterday's CAT scan showed a spot on your lung and, though it is hopefully nothing, she cannot be sure. It can be observed and reexamined in three months or biopsied now. Since it is unclear what is best, she leaves it up to you. You choose to have a biopsy. You also decide to stop smoking. *Health care includes choice.*

An hour later the nurse comes in with your medicines. When you ask why one of them is different from what you take at home, he tells you that the hospital has a contract with a company that makes this less expensive one. You are not comfortable with the change and ask for what you usually take. He promises to tell his supervisor about your concern. Health care is expensive, making cost controls and standardization of services a required part of sound business practice. *Health care is an industry.*

Around 10:00 a.m. a specialist arrives to explain the biopsy procedure. He spends very little time talking to you, instead putting information into the electronic medical record on his portable computer. You've noticed that doctors are spending more time looking at computer screens and less time talking to you.[9] New demands for data require electronic record keeping so that performance measures can be documented and new reporting requirements met. *Health care needs to be a measurable and efficient system.*

After he leaves, the nurse's aide comes by to ask you if you are comfortable, if you are getting the food you ordered, if you need help going to the bathroom, and if your family is coming by to visit soon. This personal touch makes a big difference in how you feel. *Health care is caring.*

After lunch, an administrator pays a visit. Unfortunately, if you want your usual medicine, you will need to pay the one-thousand-dollar difference, since your insurance will not cover it. You remember the problems you had last year when you had no health insurance— you couldn't afford to pay for your diabetes and high blood pressure medicine, and you had a stroke. You decide to be grateful for the medicine the insurance does cover. *Health care is a safety net with many holes.*

The reason you have health insurance now is that after your disabling stroke, you were eligible for a government program that was unavailable when you were healthy. If a new law currently under debate is passed, being disabled won't be necessary to get this insurance. You think of your uninsured friends with chronic illness and hope they vote for approval. *Health care depends on politics.*

In the afternoon, after your biopsy, someone from the public health department comes in. Your doctor heard you wanted to stop smoking and solicited the support of those involved in a new smoking cessation program. After looking at the data, they saw that smoking, along with obesity, was contributing to a large amount of disease in the community. Dedicated personnel have been trained to help people to be healthier. *Health care includes prevention and has social and community impact.*

The following morning your doctor has some concerning news— the biopsy was positive for cancer. You feel overwhelmed by the diagnosis and break down in tears. Your doctor knows you well from years of caring for you and your family. She listens to your concerns, asks if you want her to be present when you tell your husband and daughter, and carefully answers your questions. You trust her and tell her that you are afraid of dying and never seeing your unborn grandchild. She assures you that she will be with you every step of the way. You are comforted that you will share this experience with someone who knows you intimately. *Health care can be a sacred encounter of vulnerability and trust.*

Health as Possession or Health as Gift

Each face of health care has a unique perspective on what health care should be. But like carnival mirrors at an amusement park, their individual views distort the image. For health care to be good, we need the pieces to fit together. But our image of health care, giving proper place and proportion to each piece, depends on our understanding of health. And this—at its most basic level—begins with an important question: Is health a possession or a gift? The answer makes all the difference.

If health is a possession, it is *my* health—something to have and hold, a thing like any other substantive reality, such as money, cars, or houses. It is a good definable in my own terms and, as a material value, obtainable at whatever level our societal resources and my individual purchasing abilities allow. Health like this depends on choice—which makes having many choices essential. Coinciding with this view of health is a strong trend to make health care a commodity and the patient a consumer who chooses among a menu of options to control health. This is the expanding world for much of health care today. As long as we remain here, we are in danger that our worries will increase, our wasteful spending will multiply, and our waylaid commitments to neighbor will become wanton disregard.

But now consider another way, where health is received as a gift. Rather than seeing health as a material good managed for our personal happiness, we receive it as a precious endowment. What would that mean for why we pursue health and how we shape health care?

First, endowments are not given in equal portions; therefore, health will not be received in equal amounts. This is verified by our everyday experiences; some are born with longevity in their genes and strength in their bodies, while others struggle almost daily with disability and disease. If we begin in different places, this necessarily means that there is no abstract ideal of health. Rather than pursuing perfect health, we will nurture the health we have received. In addition, we will create health care in ways that strengthen what we have been given instead of reaching for what we do not have or tightly grasping what we cannot keep.

Second, as we increasingly see health as a gift, we become better able to discern its deeper reason—it is given for a purpose, to accomplish some good beyond itself, even specific things with which we have been entrusted. It is not protected for its own sake or hoarded for fear of losing it. Instead, we nurture it so that we can use it to gain and grow other goods and benefits. We may even go so far as to see a relationship between the proportion of health we have received and the purposes we are meant to accomplish.

This is an ambitious set of assertions and will force us to grapple with many complex issues. What do we do when the endowment seems small? How do we respond when our endowment is diminished through bad choice, bad luck, bad care, or all of these? Or when we risk our investment and experience loss, or our health diminishes as a part of aging? Acknowledging that there are a multitude of factors along the way that can alter our health, the view of health as gift appreciates the value of good health care. The maintenance of health and prevention and treatment of disease—endeavors we have begun to grasp with increasing clarity and success—will be sound goals when reasonably and wisely pursued. But if we lose track of what health is for, our personal pursuits will remain selfish and unsatisfied, and our health care systems will continue to grow in fragmented, irrational, and unjust ways.

The Corruption of the Best Is the Worst

"The corruption of the best is the worst" is a proverb found in many forms, from Aristotle to Aquinas to Shakespeare, but never more quaintly phrased than by English poet John Denham: "'Tis the most certain sign the world's accurst, that the best things corrupted are the worst."[10] A basic premise of this book is that health is one of those things. It is a good, one of our highest goods. But like most goods that are gifts, our efforts to insure, guarantee, or possess it will corrupt it. Like the intimate love of a spouse, the loyalty of a faithful friend, or the satisfaction of doing work well, health grows when we nurture it but diminishes when we try to control it. In the pages that follow, we will seek to renew our view of health in the hope that we can make better sense of the health we have, the sickness we experience, and the death we must inevitably face. We will divide our endeavor into four parts.

The first part sketches the basic features of our newfound faith in the capacity to control our health. We have traveled a long distance from our predecessors in the age-old challenge of living with sickness and death. Our embrace of individualism, trust in science, and extraordinary expectations of technology have fueled a fanciful hope that we can construct our own safe reality. But it was not that way at the beginning.

In the second part, we will search for the place of the person in the formation of good and just health care. Current medical practice is at risk of losing the person while pursuing health—either by reducing people to a set of functioning and fixable parts or by limiting them to their predictable behaviors as an average member of a statistically defined population. To keep the person in his or her rightful place, we need a view of people that exceeds our usual perceptions.

In the third part, we will look directly at the greatest fear in life—death. When we turn to health care—both mainline and alternative—to overcome death, our excessive expectations turn them into bloated and dysfunctional systems. In contrast to a closed view of life that restricts our hope for immortality to the here and now stands a pivotal event in human history—the resurrection of Jesus Christ from the dead. If this life is not all there is, then how we pursue health and form medicine will be drastically different.

In the last part, we will apply a redeemed view of health to two current challenges. First, we will ask if understanding health as gift can lead to a wider sharing and a more just distribution of health care to those who need it most. Finally we will explore the frayed connections between faith and medicine. Though the current milieu has encouraged their separation, it will be worth exploring the underlying connections that bind them together for the sake of better health.

The Hope for Health

1

Taking Control of Health

The Need to Feel Invulnerable

Humpty Dumpty sat on a wall,
Humpty Dumpty had a great fall;
All the king's horses and all the king's men
Couldn't put Humpty together again.

Nursery rhymes are useful for a number of reasons. First, they rhyme, which makes them easy to remember. But they can also carry a great deal of meaning. One of the most familiar in the English language, Humpty Dumpty is usually represented as an anthropomorphic egg. Why is he up on that wall when all he has to protect him is his fragile shell?

But Humpty, if we can be informal, doesn't feel vulnerable. In fact, his response to Alice in Lewis Carroll's *Through the Looking-Glass* suggests he is quite comfortable. When Alice suggests Humpty would be safer on the ground, he is smug and unconcerned. He's not afraid of falling. And if he did—though he never would—he knows the king, who has promised all the strength and power at his disposal. Humpty may not be a good egg, as we will see, but he is a confident one.

Carroll's expansion of the rhyme reveals another side of Humpty. Secure in his place on the wall, he assumes the power to choose the meaning of words, one of them being *glory*:

> "I don't know what you mean by 'glory,'" Alice said.
>
> Humpty Dumpty smiled contemptuously. "Of course you don't—till I tell you. I meant 'there's a nice knock-down argument for you!'"
>
> "But 'glory' doesn't mean 'a nice knock-down argument,'" Alice objected.
>
> "When I use a word," Humpty Dumpty said, in rather a scornful tone, "it means just what I choose it to mean—neither more nor less."
>
> "The question is," said Alice, "whether you *can* make words mean so many different things."
>
> "The question is," said Humpty Dumpty, "which is to be master—that's all."[1]

Eventually tiring of his pompous attitude, Alice soon walks away. Muttering to herself, "of all the unsatisfactory people I *ever* met—"[2] her thoughts are suddenly interrupted by a loud crash that shakes the forest from end to end. As we know, things didn't turn out well for Humpty. Despite all the king's help, it was not enough to put him back together.

Aren't We Like Him?

Though we prefer not to think about it, we are very much like Humpty Dumpty. In spite of our own fragile shells, we believe we can sit safely on the precarious wall of life. Although our world is full of disease, accidents, and random misfortunes, many of us never plan on being sick or dying and are quite shocked when we are. How have we come to think like *that* in a world like *this*?

Again, we can look to Humpty, seeing what helps him feel invulnerable. First, he lives in a fairy tale, where assumptions are not tested because reality is not fixed. Second, in the freedom of his fantasy world, he has come to believe that his thin shell is thick enough to protect him. Lastly, he has gained great confidence from making his own meaning for things.

Haven't we arrived at our own sense of invulnerability by depending on the same things? We live in a kind of fairy tale world, don't we? Certain ideas, though fantasy, are taken for granted simply by breathing in the air of our age. We, too, have come to believe that we live in a shell thick enough to buffer us from the dangers around us. And we have found it very helpful to make our own meaning for things.

Upon this foundation of invulnerability we have rested our belief that we can control our health. Let's look at the components of this structure more carefully.

The Air We Breathe

In my childhood home, there were certain things we believed and did without thinking. No one questioned, for example, why we always had turkey for Christmas—even though we had all ceased liking it long ago. We still considered our neighbor Mr. Barney to be a grumpy old man and avoided him—even though he hadn't been mean to kids for twenty years. Though our rationales were long gone, we took for granted the way things were.

Similar to a childhood home, though more confusing and complex, we are also raised in a cultural home containing many assumptions. Constructed over hundreds of years with many builders but no master plan, one of its most pervasive assumptions is that we can flourish without any help from God. Philosopher Charles Taylor, in his book *A Secular Age*, carefully defines this space as the "immanent frame,"[3] a space we share with all who have been brought up in the modern world with a Western mind-set:[4]

> The great invention of the West was that of an immanent order in Nature, whose working could be systematically understood and explained on its own terms. . . . This notion of the "immanent" involved denying—or at least isolating and problematizing—any form of interpenetration between the things of Nature, on the one hand, and "the supernatural" on the other, be this understood in

terms of the one transcendent God, or of Gods or spirits, or magic forces, or whatever.[5]

Inside the enclosure of the immanent frame that separates the spiritual world from the material world, we can find fullness within human life, so the underlying assumptions of our age declare.

The reactions to this reality are variable. Some deny any influence of this assumption in their lives.[6] Some fully embrace it, installing a brass ceiling on their immanent frame. Others put in skylights, gaining purpose and meaning through these intermittent openings to the transcendent.[7] But none escape its effects. All unconsciously breathe in the air of the age. Operating powerfully and silently in the background of our mind, each of us is affected by the cultural idea that we can flourish on our own terms.

As outside observers of a comic-strip world, watch for the hidden assumption in a conversation between Rat and Goat one Sunday morning in *Pearls Before Swine*.[8] Goat informs Rat that his forty-two-year-old neighbor Fred suddenly died. Rat wonders why and asks what high-risk health behavior could have caused his death. Was he overweight? Did he smoke? Were there family members with heart disease? None of these were true, which made Rat very nervous. Maybe he used drugs or drove super-fast motorcycles in the rain? But he didn't do any of those things. Rat is now frantic—if Fred died suddenly and didn't do any of those things, Rat realizes it could happen to him. "Give me something about Fred that made him different than me!" Rat implores. "He collected stamps," Goat replies. "High-risk hobby. He was doomed," concludes Rat, relaxing again in his fantastic but comforting assumption that every death has an obvious cause and, if we know what it is, we can prevent it.[9]

Though humorous, it exposes the powerful influence of the immanent frame, especially prominent in our view of health and sickness. If all that matters is human flourishing, and if all that is needed for humans to flourish can be found within human life, then each sickness, accident, and death includes the assumption that it is unnecessary and avoidable.

Even behind a strong religious faith we can see the silent assumption at work. A friend of mine once cared for a pastor who had a debilitating stroke at age seventy-two. He was bound to a wheelchair for years after, and his wife struggled with why God would allow this to happen to her husband, a devoted man who had served God all his life. His good life should have gained him a safe place on the wall of this world. Somehow the idea that life can be controlled to our satisfaction by a mixture of good behavior, good choices, good medicine, or a good God—if he does what we expect—enters into the pores of our being without our notice. So strongly do we take these things for granted that when we meet someone who doesn't, it confuses us.

When Ellen was diagnosed with ovarian cancer at age sixty-two, her friends could not understand it. She had worked for years in Christian service to the poor and homeless in Washington, DC. "Why would God allow something like this to happen to a person like you?" they asked her. "Why not me?" she responded, only increasing their perplexity in her refusal to accept their assumption. For Ellen knew what many do not realize—that a world where humans can flourish apart from God and control the circumstances of their lives is no different from Humpty's world; it is a fantasy.

The Shell of the Buffered Self

To further our sense of invulnerability, like Humpty, we need a novel way of thinking about ourselves. Humpty Dumpty had an "attitude," I'm sure Alice would concur, a peculiar perception of himself that enabled him to feel invulnerable despite the narrow wall upon which he sat and the fragile shell within which he lived. We have developed an attitude as well, though it has taken a long while to get there—not surprising since it is in such marked contrast to where we started. Over the course of five hundred years we have developed what Taylor calls a "buffered self."[10]

In the world of the 1500s, he explains, our medieval ancestors saw the cosmos as an untamed spirit world of light and darkness, good and bad, order and chaos. People felt vulnerable, "porous,"[11] to the field of forces around them. Observing the random nature of accidents, illnesses, and other misfortunes, they assumed that their lives could be shattered at any moment. Naturally, people sought refuge in their social world, embedding themselves in a network of communal relationships that gave support and protection. At the same time, belief in God as the dominant spirit amongst many was a great assurance that unpredictable forces would not freely gallop into their lives and wreak havoc. Living without God in the scary world of our medieval ancestors was hardly an option.

Before advancing to the modern solution, it is worth remembering that many of our global neighbors still retain a porous view of reality. In many traditional cultures, it is believed that random forces—affecting everything from weather changes to crop failures to sickness and death—are always at work. The only way to organize life with any sense of control is to populate it with spiritual forces that are known and placatable. When I was working in central Africa, one of my patients died from a ruptured aortic aneurysm, a sudden and unfortunate event. From my perspective, there was no one to blame or any treatment that would have saved him. But many in the family had a different understanding. Years before his death, when he was studying abroad, he failed to attend the funeral of his father. This offended his father's spirit, they said, and that is why he died. While this culture depended on ancestors to intervene, others believe that members of the community possess special powers. Although some trust in one God, many find a pantheon of gods more reassuring. Whatever the mix, the goal is always the same—to gain a sense of control in a random world.

We in the modern West are no different. We too desire control, but with expectations that make depending on God or a spirit world far too unreliable. So we have replaced a cosmos of spirits and forces with a mechanistic universe of predictable patterns.[12] And then for what remains unpredictable, unpleasant, or uncomfortable, we have added the boundary of the buffered self. It lies between our internal thinking selves and the external world—a wall separating inside and outside that is our shell.[13] Within this buffered self we are able to disengage from anything outside the mind that disturbs us. Inside my shell, nothing need "get to me." Now, like Humpty, we can feel invulnerable.[14] All that's left is to make our thoughts the master of meaning.

The Power to Construct Our Own Meaning

At the same time that the mechanization of the universe made the natural world more predictable, it also drained it of any inherent meaning. From planets that orbit the sun to birds that migrate south, the universe is now akin to a ticking clock, each part performing its perfunctory function in perfect obedience to the laws of nature, with no meaning or purpose beyond its programmed utility.

With the external world emptied of its own meaning, meaning-seeking creatures like us are free to impose it, making each one of us the author of meaning. Taylor calls this "self-authorization."[15] He writes, "My ultimate purposes are those which arise within me, the crucial meaning of things are those defined in my responses to them. . . . This self can see itself as invulnerable, as master of the meaning of things for it."[16] Or, as Humpty would say, "When I use a word, it means just what I choose it to mean—neither more nor less."

Humpty was merely an egg ahead of his time. For as French philosopher Alain Renaut describes it, self-authorization has become a central feature of modernity:

> What constitutes modernity is the fact that man thinks of himself as the source of his representations and acts, as their foundation (subject) or their author. . . . The man of humanism is the one who no longer receives his norms and laws either from the nature of things (Aristotle) or from God, but who establishes them himself on the basis of his reason and will.[17]

The autonomous power to determine our own meaning has permitted the idea of "health control" to take deeper root in our cultural home. Not limited by any external source, we are free to make our own way and determine our own happiness. But each one seeking his or her own meaning apart from any external standard or limit can also be a heavy burden—and not a small source of confusion and pain, in our common struggle to know who we are and where we belong.

Have It Your Way

But wasn't Humpty Dumpty right? The most important thing is "to be master—that's all." As buffered, self-authorizing individuals, we can order our world and flourish on our own terms. With each his or her own master, and freedom of choice the prime value, we can have it the way we want it.[18]

And so we arrive at the dominant individualism of our age, "in which people are encouraged to find their own way, discover their own fulfillment, 'do their own thing.'"[19] Catalyzed by the merger of individual choice with the consumer culture of post-war affluence, each person and every aspect of society has now been marked by the "have it your way" mentality.[20] In health care and medicine, it may have infiltrated more slowly but no less effectively.

To be sure, a good portion of health care has resisted these forces and remains a straightforward and commonly accepted action for a clear and present problem—surgery for appendicitis, a cast for a broken bone, or an antibiotic to treat pneumonia. In these situations of immediate threat, the standard treatment for many conditions offers a high likelihood of success in protecting life and restoring health. We accept these blessings of modern medicine with little hesitation. Who would choose otherwise?

But in the last thirty years we have seen an unprecedented growth of health care in areas heretofore considered outside the jurisdiction of medicine and increasingly dependent on choice; an obvious example is the aging category, with components such as balding and decreased sexual function. As the line between normal and pathologic is increasingly blurred and benefits become less obvious, individual choice—the prime good of self-authorization—becomes more prominent. Freedom of choice in health care is the most rapidly growing part of twenty-first-century medicine. Yet it is not the unadulterated good it may seem when first faced with an array of options.

Conception and pregnancy care have been a particular focus of revolutionary change. Starting with the array of treatments for infertility, there has been an explosion of choices—some in your body (in vivo), some outside it (in vitro), and some using another body (surrogacy). Once pregnant, prenatal testing—unheard of when I first began to offer obstetrical care in the 1980s[21]—offers further options for managing your pregnancy, as Joyce and Samuel discovered when they went to their first prenatal visit. While current prenatal testing focuses on a healthy baby at birth, future options will look further out, measuring risks that would only occur much later in life and with much less certainty. New methods under investigation can inform you that your future child has 1.5 percent risk of developing schizophrenia as a young adult, above the usual 1 percent risk; or that fifty years from now your baby will have an increased risk of developing colon cancer.[22] As the information becomes increasingly ambiguous and the possible outcomes more distant, the freedom of choice turns into a burden of options, creating anxious parents-to-be who don't know what to do with the information they have.[23]

Many of these changes in modern medicine are driven by the desires of the autonomous self-authorizing individual—full of choice, a focus on future possibilities over current disease, and an emphasis on improving the given model over maintaining or regaining basic health. In short, modern medicine looks increasingly more like the pursuit of happiness and control of the future than the cure of sickness and the care of health.

What If We Fall?

Humpty Dumpty has taught us a lot about ourselves. He sat on a high wall with nothing to protect him but a thin eggshell; we live in an unpredictable and often hostile world with nothing but our fragile bodies. Despite these realities, we too have learned to feel invulnerable. His self-delusion is the result of living in a fairy tale; ours is the result of living in a fantasy age, where health is a controllable commodity and meaning is a personal choice for interpretation.

But, like Humpty, we still need a contingency plan. Necessary to solidify our view of health as within our control, we need something akin to a powerful king as our ally; after all, if we fall, we might get hurt. Blessed to live in the age of science, we are trusting in the techniques of medicine to rescue us. Though the king's resources weren't enough to save Humpty, the promises of science are different, more reliable than horses and men—and if more reliable, then better able to put us back together, we presume. But putting the pieces together and keeping us whole is harder than we realize.

In the next chapter we will consider these questions as we evaluate the role of science in our lives. Confidently expecting a sure rescue if ever we fall off the wall, we are in danger of placing excessive faith in science, corrupting it by the very overreach we are asking of it. If we have any hope of regaining wholeness in our quest for healing, we need to determine the good and proper place of science.

2

The Desire for Certainty
in an Uncertain World

The greater our medical successes, the more unacceptable is failure, and the more frightening and intolerable is death.

Leon Kass

Not long ago I took a long walk in an old cemetery in the capital city of New Zealand. I do this sometimes when visiting a new place. It reminds me how far we have come, yet how fundamentally fragile life is. Tombstones tell stories in the most abbreviated form but rich with memory and meaning. Two in particular stood out that day.

On one stone were the names of five children. At the end of December 1876, in the short span of eleven days, their parents watched helplessly as each one, all less than twelve years old, died from diphtheria. Today diphtheria is a rare disease thanks to a vaccine—in 2013 most countries, including the United States, had no cases.[1]

A little distance further was a tombstone with the names of three children, also from a single family. Over a one-month period, in the same year as the children in the other family, scarlet fever came and took their young lives, at the ages of three, four, and five. In 1993, when my son was four years old, he had scarlet fever. Quickly diagnosed and treated, he was feeling better in three days. Because of a simple course of antibiotics, only a little more than one hundred years later, my family was spared the tragedy of these other families.

How far we have come and how fortunate we are to live in this age of advanced medical science.

The Fruits of Science

Achievements in the sciences have produced great benefits for humankind, reducing or removing many of the terrors that defined the lives of our ancestors. Bubonic plague decimated Europe in the fourteenth century. Happening before the discovery of bacteriology, no one understood its cause or could prescribe a program to control its course. We have now eradicated smallpox and nearly removed the scourge of polio. A swine flu epidemic can still engender fear today, yet the mechanisms that define its propagation are quickly evaluated, and a program of prevention and treatment rapidly restricts its effects.

The control of infectious diseases clearly represents one of the greatest benefits of applied science for the betterment of humankind. Public health measures that prevent disease, such as those that defined and limited the spread of cholera in England in the 1800s, have likely had the larger effect. Yet the ability to diagnose, treat, and cure already infected individuals, saving them from death, brightly shines in our collective consciousness as the model of medicinal power. In the early 1900s the major infectious diseases, with no curative treatment, filled hospital beds and carried off patients with depressing regularity.[2] The discovery of penicillin in 1928, and its broad application to sick soldiers during the Second World War, changed bacterial pneumonia from the "captain of the men of death" to a treatable condition.[3] Today even a few days to recover at home or in a hospital disrupt our busy lives, while before modern treatments it often meant the end of life.

The power found within the scientific method of observation and experimentation to establish "cause and effect" has profoundly changed our relationship with nature. Much of what was chaotic and uncontrollable, from infectious disease to heart disease, from leukemia to diabetes, has become amenable to investigation and control. But a danger constantly lurks that we will assume all reality can succumb to this power.

The Rationale for Optimism in Medical Science

The age of science ushered in by the Enlightenment began a new chapter in humanity's relationship with nature. Up to that point, truth about the natural world heavily depended on the thought of antiquity and the written authority of traditionally valued books.[4] Natural philosophies taught the observation and admiration of nature's overall pattern but did little in the way of its investigation and control.

But practitioners of the new philosophy of science, notables such as William Harvey, whose experiments in the early 1600s led to the correct understanding of how blood circulates in the body,[5] preferred the study of a different text, the book of nature. They saw potent knowledge available to any bold enough to examine a book so open for consultation.[6] Most of these early scientists initially understood the laws of nature as written into creation by the hand of God.[7] Some even made sure the laws stayed subject to God's pleasure, so that "it should be understood that stones fell downward, at thirty-two feet per second squared, *God willing.*"[8] But the idea that God's will was greater than God's reason progressively gave way to more and more dependence on human reason and less and less need for God, leading to what Charles Taylor has aptly called "exceptionless natural law" functioning unalterably in an "impersonal order."[9]

Consider the benefits of such a worldview. With nature this predictable, and a methodology of science able to unlock its secrets through demonstrable, repeatable, and reliable investigation, there is no limit to the control of nature for the betterment of humankind.[10] At the beginning of the twentieth century, on the heels of the stunning triumphs of medical science up to that time, including Rudolph Virchow's discovery of the cell, Louis Pasteur's discovery of bacteriology, and Joseph Lister's use of sterile procedure that made the

operating room a safe place, optimistic faith in medical science was
nearly boundless.

Man's Redemption of Man

William Osler was one of the most admired and honored physicians
in the history of medicine. The span of his life, 1849–1919, bridged
the achievements of the nineteenth century with the anticipation of the
twentieth century. Toward the end of his illustrious career in 1910,
reflecting on the advance of science and all that lay ahead, he delivered
an address he entitled "Man's Redemption of Man."[11]

Delivered to 2,500 listeners at the University of Edinburgh, he
spoke glowingly of the achievements of nineteenth-century medicine.
With the rise of the scientific spirit in modern times, it was his belief
that with the help of men like Charles Darwin, who has "so turned
man right-about-face that, no longer looking back with regret upon
a Paradise Lost, he feels already within the gates of a Paradise Re-
gained,"[12] medical scientists would redeem humanity from pain, fever,
and disease. Using repeated biblical allusions to a new heaven and a
new earth, in each case he saw the fruits of science accomplishing here
and now what was anticipated in Scripture. Seeing that "the leaves
of the tree of science have availed for the healing of the nations," he
glowingly described the discovery of anesthesia:

> On October 16, 1846, in the amphitheater of Massachusetts Gen-
> eral Hospital, Boston, a new Prometheus gave a gift as rich as that
> of fire, the greatest single gift ever made to suffering humanity.
> The prophecy was fulfilled—*neither shall there be any more pain*;
> a mystery of the ages has been solved by a daring experiment by
> man on man in the introduction of anesthesia. . . . At a stroke the
> curse of Eve was removed.[13]

Believing that the outlook for the world had never been so hopeful,
he ended his address with eager anticipation of the glorious day envi-
sioned by English Romantic poet Percy Bysshe Shelley:

> Happiness
> And Science dawn though late upon the earth;

Peace cheers the mind, health renovates the frame;
Disease and pleasure cease to mingle here,
Reason and passion cease to combat there,
Whilst mind unfettered o'er the earth extends
Its all-subduing energies, and wields
The sceptre of a vast dominion there.[14]

These were truly heady times in the history of medicine. In many ways the next one hundred years went a long way to fulfilling the hopes and dreams of this moment—lucky for Humpty, who was more prone to falling than he realized.

Before the Big Fall

Reason suggests that Humpty took his lumps, falling several times before the big one. Let's consider a few of his other accidents. First, it was because of his imperfect genes. He was born a little lopsided—not a perfect oval—though he would never admit it, which required him to pay attention when he got up to do his daily exercise on the wall. One day, he got distracted, forgot to compensate, and fell. Another time, it was just bad luck—a gust of wind at the wrong time. And what about that time he got in an argument with his resentful neighbor—not a Grade A Jumbo egg like Humpty but only medium grade—who came up behind and pushed him.

Each time the damage was reparable, thanks to the advances of medical science. The orthopedic doctors pinned the broken bones in his arm after the first fall. The second time he fell on his side and lacerated his kidney, but the surgeons were able to stop the bleeding. It was more dangerous when he hit his head after being pushed by his neighbor; fortunately it was only a subdural hematoma, and the neurosurgeons drained it. Each time he recovered under the watchful eye of the highly skilled medical team. It was particularly difficult after his brain injury; he was getting older, after all, and he had been recently diagnosed with diabetes. But after two weeks in the intensive care unit and two more weeks in a regular unit, he was able to go back to his wall. Each time they sent him back, he was a little more wobbly than before—until that final fall when, no matter how hard they tried, they couldn't put him back together.

Medicine's Failure, or Recalcitrant Realities

If we experience repeated successes after we fall, success becomes routine, and our expectations rise that every time we fall, we will get better; we even convince ourselves that what people died from yesterday won't be fatal tomorrow, as medical science continues to advance, conquering new territory every day. William Osler was right—with enough time and energy and money, we will eventually "relieve the human condition of the human condition,"[15] realizing the biblical promises here and now.

But then the day comes when the incurable happens. It could be cancer, it could be heart disease, it could be a simple fall but at an older age—this time the pieces just won't go back together. In almost every case, at some point there is a sense of failure—for the patient, for the family, and for the health care team.

Not long ago a journalist for the *Los Angeles Times* died after a long struggle with breast cancer. She wrote of her journey with particular poignancy, contributing installments until her last days. She had lived for many years with cancer. But as the days wound down, with all known therapies exhausted, she was understandably frustrated as the disease progressed. Not unusually, she blamed the system. In an op-ed, published after her death, she wrote, "The medical establishment tells me I have 'failed' a number of therapies. That's not right: The establishment and its therapies have failed me."[16]

Feeling that the medical system has failed is an increasingly common reaction when problems aren't fixed or diseases aren't cured. No area of medicine can escape this sense of failure. Most obvious is oncology, when it involves incurable cancer. But rheumatologists cannot cure lupus, cardiologists still lose patients after a heart attack, neurologists must help people live with disability after a stroke, and even dermatologists see some patients die from melanoma. In every case there is a sense of failure, for both the patient and the profession. I remember a young couple who were distraught after enduring their third miscarriage. How is it, the husband asked, that the medical profession can do so little to prevent this from happening? All I could do was share their sense of impotence.[17]

We cannot help but be discomforted by these tragic experiences.

At the very least they remind us we are vulnerable, despite the best efforts of our buffered selves to assure us we are not. At times we are angry and feel that the promise of medicine has failed us. But science and technology are bound to fail if we ask them to fulfill promises of biblical proportions. What we often miss are the downsides of our delusion: a corruption of the very science we depend on to achieve our grandiose goals, the narrowing of reality to solvable problems, and an increasing fear of what remains uncertain, no matter how small that is.

The Corruption of Science in Our Quest for Control

Erwin Chargaff, a renowned scientist whose research into the chemical composition of nucleic acids laid the groundwork for the discovery of the DNA molecule, believed in the grandeur of science. In his memoir, *Heraclitean Fire*, he offered several ways to measure its greatness:

> If it is the real purpose of science to teach us true things about nature, to reveal to us the reality of the world, the consequence of such teaching ought to be increased wisdom, a greater love of nature, and, in a few, a heightened admiration of divine power. By confronting us directly with something greater than ourselves, science should serve to push back the confines of the misery of human existence.[18]

As a scientist trained in the experimental method, he rigorously pursued the investigation of nature, hoping to reduce "the misery of human existence" as part of the good purpose of science. But he saw in the confines of his research community of the mid-twentieth century a progressive distortion of science as it was applied for greater and greater control. From "an undertaking designed to understand nature, it has changed into one attempting to explain, and then improve, on nature."[19] With an overemphasis on the mechanical side, the focus had turned to making "the postulated wheels and gears operate to produce presupposed effects and to reach posited goals."[20]

In reducing things to the manipulation of mechanical parts for our intended ends, we gain power and control; the double helix of DNA becomes a "spiral stairway leading into heaven,"[21] reminiscent of William Osler's faith that science applied to humanity's problems would regain paradise. But reductive science, though it gives us useful tools, forces things into simplified forms, even distorting reality to make it fit the mold. Chargaff went so far as to call this overuse of the scientific method a "bulldozer of reality":[22]

> One of the most insidious and nefarious properties of scientific models is their tendency to take over, and sometimes supplant, reality. They often act as blinkers, limiting attention to an excessively narrow region. . . . The extravagant reliance on models has contributed much to the contrived and artificial character of large portions of current research.[23]

But we cannot help our fascination with tools that, when taken in hand and applied, turn the screw and fit the nut to produce the intended result. Everyone likes a simple problem with a direct solution, even if it does distort reality.

The Paradigm of Problem and Solution

Odd as it may sound, many of my colleagues, myself included, like treating sexually transmitted diseases—because for most we have a curative "magic bullet" in our toolbox. But initial satisfaction at having a specific treatment for a known condition quickly disappears when faced with the deeper cause—someone's unfaithfulness that exposed the patient to the infection in the first place. So much dis-ease remains after the antibiotic is swallowed or the injection given. Was the patient unfaithful and now feels guilty, or denies it because it is too painful to admit? Or did her husband wander away, and now she cries out, hoping there is someone who will mourn with her over broken relationships that destroy families faster than the plague?

Though deeper realities get bulldozed aside, the myth of the scientific project persistently begs for further application, preferentially using the way we achieved success in infectious disease as the operating model for all of life's problems. If we can link a causative agent similar to a virus or bacteria to each and every problem, then science can apply its methods and discover a fixable cause and final solution for each and every effect. Though satisfying when it works, it fashions an incomplete vision of reality.

To reduce most moments in life to a scientific simplicity of problem then solution is language, English writer and scholar Dorothy Sayers suggests, that is misleading:

> It is here that we begin to see how the careless use of the words "problem" and "solution" can betray us into habits of thought that are not merely inadequate but false. It leads us to consider all vital activities in terms of a particular kind of problem, namely the kind we associate with elementary mathematics and detective fiction. . . . Applied indiscriminately, they are fast becoming a deadly danger. They falsify our apprehension of life as disastrously as they falsify our apprehension of art.[24]

As a detective fiction writer herself, she knew full well that the writer so constructs the mystery to permit readers a single satisfactory solution if they but persist to the end. Sayers saw this pleasing outcome as the reason for the extraordinary popularity of this genre of literature in her time.[25] It offers a modern understanding of mystery, as a puzzle that can be solved, rather than a reality that must be embraced.

In our desire to "solve life" we continue to reduce the mystery of birth, sickness, and death into controllable categories. We even get frustrated with the idea that these kinds of things would escape the boxes we put them in, as Sayers suggests:

> From very early days, alchemists have sought the elixir of life, so reluctant is man to concede that there can be any problem incapable of a solution. And of late, we note a growing resentment and exasperation in the face of death. . . . Our efforts are not directed, like those of the saint or the poet, to make something creative out of the idea of death, but rather to seeing whether we cannot somehow evade, abolish, and, in fact, "solve the problem" of death.[26]

But demanding certainty for uncertain events will always distort. Consider the side effects of our efforts to "solve" the uncertainty of birth, an event that has always been one of the most uncertain in life, until recently. Gratefully, much has been done to secure the health and safety of newborn life. Historically, having children was a huge gamble. As recently as 1915, one in every ten children born in the United States died by the first year of life. By 2012 that number was one in 160, changing the experience of pregnancy from naturally risky to almost always safe.[27]

Having highly reasonable hopes of survival has been a great achievement and wonderful blessing. But on top of these benefits of modern science, new layers of expectations are added. Not satisfied with a high likelihood of a healthy birth, we want the outcome certain, the baby perfect, and maybe even the delivery at a convenient time. But the demand for certainty is an intolerant master, unnecessarily forcing many births into operative procedures.

When first measured in 1965, 4.5 percent of all children born in the United States were delivered by caesarean section.[28] In 2009 that number had risen to almost 33 percent,[29] making one of every three pregnancies an operative delivery, each one with higher cost and the added complications of surgery. The rate has remained similar in subsequent years, despite recommendations that it is much too high. Among the many reasons that contribute to this excessive rate,[30] several of the most important factors show up in a typical day for any obstetrician.

Dr. Booth has just finished a scheduled caesarean section. Her patient had had this operation for her first pregnancy, and when they discussed natural labor for the second, though recommended and safe to try, it seemed easier to opt for the certainty of a planned operation. Soon after, Dr. Booth is called to the room of a patient in labor because the fetal heart rate is slowing with her contractions. She tells her patient that these changes are not specific for any problems and recommends observation. But the patient, afraid her baby is not getting enough oxygen, wants a caesarean section. Dr. Booth thinks it is better to wait, but then she remembers a conversation with Dr. Lee earlier that day in the doctors' lounge. He is being sued by one of his patients whose child was born with respiratory problems. Wasn't that case just like this? Thinking of how often obstetricians are being sued for malpractice, she agrees to do the operation. Later that day as she reflects on her decisions, she wonders how it happened. Whether questionable fetal heart tracings or the unknowns of labor after a prior caesarean section, in a potent mix with physician fear of liability, the natural process of childbirth is now a dangerous event. She never thought obstetrics would be like that.

But maybe more operations and higher costs are just the price we have to pay in our quest for greater control over the birth of our babies? And more technology when we are fighting death is another necessity we have to accept. But why do greater certainty and more control only heighten our fear for what remains outside our control—especially if the possibilities are so improbable?

A Greater Fear of Unlikely Occurrences

In one of the lesser-known travels of Gulliver, author Jonathan Swift brings him to the floating island of Laputa. He finds that the people of this land have an advanced knowledge of science. But with a particular interest in astronomy, they are also in constant fear of the end of the world through some unlikely cosmic event. They know that comets hit the earth, so they worry that the next time will be a direct hit and reduce them to ashes. Or, observing the orbit of the earth around the sun, they fear that one day the earth will be swallowed up into it. So sure the shoe is going to drop at any minute, they are unable to enjoy any of the pleasantness of their lives.

> These People are under continual Disquietudes, never enjoying a Minute's Peace of Mind; and their Disturbances proceed from Causes which very little affect the rest of Mortals. Their Apprehensions arise from several Changes they dread in the Celestial Bodies. . . . They are so perpetually alarmed with the Apprehensions of these and the like impending Dangers, that they can neither sleep quietly in their Beds, nor have any relish for the common Pleasures or Amusements of Life.[31]

Writing in the early 1700s as the age of science was stretching its muscles, Swift, one of the greatest of English satirists, was allegorically describing the dangers of overdependence on science, not the least being the prediction of danger and doom when it was little if at all in sight. Though secure in a land of plenty, floating high above the problems of the rest of the world, the Laputans worried about the improbable because they knew it was possible. Much to Swift's credit, it turns out that this can be a problem for us all.

In this day and age, we may not fear the next comet (or do we?), but we do worry about something less rare: the report of an abnormal medical test. Having delivered the news on numerous occasions, it is hard to curb the anxiety created by an uncertain result. Often there is little connection between the likelihood that something bad will happen and the reaction it engenders; whether the person actually has cancer or the screening test is abnormal but the chance of cancer is extremely small, the word *cancer* is enough to turn life upside down.[32] Curiously, the more in control a person feels before the news, the more it disrupts his world. Often we find patients of lower socioeconomic status, already with limited control or predictability in life, accepting the news with little change in equilibrium. But the one whose calendar is organized for the next six months is overwhelmed with fear. Like the Laputans, the more we know and the more secure life seems, the more we fear what remains outside our control, no matter how small the likelihood.

In recent times, removing potentially dangerous body parts has become one of the more radical ways to remove uncertainty in our modern age. One example is the surgical removal of the opposite breast (contralateral prophylactic mastectomy) in patients with unilateral breast cancer. Though there are rare high-risk groups in which this may be valid, the majority of women choosing this procedure have a very low risk of cancer in the unaffected breast. Ironically, with the success of systemic therapy for breast cancer, the risk of cancer in the unaffected breast is decreasing, but the rate of bilateral mastectomy for unilateral cancer is increasing. Fear of recurrence, the intense sense of vulnerability felt by all diagnosed with cancer, and the desire to return to a peace of mind that all is secure are leading too many women to have this unnecessary surgery.[33]

Our Unique Age

At face value, we would not expect that fear would increase as danger decreases. Yet for many in our age, worry about health grows as the likelihood of sickness and death shrinks. Though the irrational power that can conjure up great fears from meager sources may be enough to explain it, let us consider a unique contribution that has come as our modern view has evolved into our late-modern perspective.

The confidence of modernity in human progress leading to continual world improvement has fallen on hard times in recent decades. For many, hope in reason and science bringing millennial fulfillment has been tempered by the excesses and evils of the twentieth century.[34] From world wars to the threat of nuclear holocaust to genocides of unspeakable horror, the many tragedies of the last one hundred years have shaken us. The world refuses to get better despite all the progress we have made.[35]

But our faith in the control wrought by science has not been discarded wholesale. In the face of persistent chaos and terror on the world stage, many of us have chosen to withdraw and restrict our efforts to the control of a smaller, more subjective world. Retreating into our buffered selves, instead of global stability we'll settle for personal control; instead of limitless possibilities for world improvement we hope for limitless possibilities of self-improvement. Though the world beyond remains unpredictable, we can still control what is close and near as the part of the world that most matters. In these later days of modernity, our demand for certainty and control hasn't changed as much as the sphere in which we expect it.

But whether we ask science to give us control of a world big and global or one small and near, godlike efforts to control our circumstances will fall short, leaving us with false hope and floating fear, as political philosopher Peter Augustine Lawler points out in his critique of individualism and biotechnology:

> The true scientific myth must actually be "Promethean"; its strength must come from giving people "blind hopes" that all that they long for can be achieved through scientific progress and liberation. The original Prometheus, Wilson remembers, "caused mortals to cease foreseeing doom." Blind hopes can cure or at least deaden the symptoms of that specifically human "sickness" of foresight.[36]

The chaos of the world has not succumbed to our "rage for order"[37] on a global scale, nor have we been able to "cease foreseeing doom" from the safety of our buffered self. Still haunted in our dreams, the best we can do is to hide the reality from our conscious selves.

In many ways we are successful with this ruse. Though Enlightenment optimism has given way to post-Enlightenment pessimism, many of us still generally know the vigor of healthy bodies; the provision of health care insurance; the assurance of food, clothing, and shelter; and a relatively peaceful town. But our peculiar preoccupations today are that there are powers lurking constantly just beyond our range of vision, waiting to break in upon us. Worst of all, we know that disaster may strike us just when we are most secure, when we have never felt better, and the phone rings to tell us our test is abnormal and we may have cancer, which we are now sure we do.

As far back as 1950, theologian Romano Guardini predicted the end of the modern age and the fear, threat, doubt, danger, and anxiety we would feel in an age he saw coming but felt unable to name:

> All monsters of the wilderness, all horrors of darkness have reappeared. The human person stands before the chaos; and all of this is so much more terrible, since the majority do not recognize it: after all, everywhere scientifically educated people are communicating with one another, machines are running smoothly, and bureaucracies are functioning well.[38]

He was far more accurate than he could have known. We may have hidden the monsters in the closet, but they are there nonetheless. And outside, in our quest for health control, we continue to hope that medical science will deliver us from the horrors of darkness that threaten us with chaos and uncertainty.

As buffered and autonomous self-authorizing creatures, we are working hard to convince ourselves that if our world is small enough, we can make it safe and secure. But our failure to accept uncertainty in life is producing a great imbalance in our health care systems. More importantly, we are misplacing our trust upon a pseudoscience that reduces all of life to mechanical functions that can be measured and controlled. But offers to make certain what are by nature contingent and mysterious realities are causing too much distortion for our own good. As poet, novelist, and cultural critic Wendell Berry suggests, we need to see the pattern of the whole that holds the pieces together and absorbs uncertainty as an essential part of who we are:

> We seem to have been living for a long time on the assumption that we can safely deal with parts, leaving the whole to take care of itself. But now the news from everywhere is that we have to begin gathering up the scattered pieces, figuring out where they belong, and putting them back together. For the parts can be reconciled to one another only within the pattern of the whole thing to which they belong.[39]

We need a view of life and health that can respond to the tragedy of cancer that fails treatment, the unfaithfulness of a spouse who has given his wife a sexually transmitted disease, or the birth of an imperfect child. We need a story that can embrace contingency without running away, even finding a way to make it meaningful. We need a "pattern of the whole thing" that accepts the basic reality that we are dependent, frail, and fragile. For that we need to go back to the beginning.

3

As It Was in the Beginning

The true God . . . will always disappoint our desire for independence and self-sufficiency.

Gilbert Meilaender

Who doesn't want autonomy and control? If we stop and think of children passing through the normal stages of development, it is only natural. At a certain point they begin to explore their world with the end of finding out how much control they can get.

Before having my own children, I first understood the basic stages of psychosocial development in my college psychology class. The most well-known process was formulated by Erik Erikson;[1] it begins with the baby's need for trust. At this stage the baby has one basic question: Is the world a safe place, or is it full of unpredictable events and accidents waiting to happen? In the setting of trustworthy care, the baby will exit this stage with the solid ground necessary for navigating the difficult quest for autonomy in the next phase of growth and development.

Beyond the textbooks, real-life experience bluntly teaches every parent the toddler's strong desire for independence; few would argue that the "terrible twos" is not aptly named. The child will test every boundary, not knowing that a healthy formation of confidence depends on a parent's wise establishment of limits. Never smooth, as every parent can attest, only within safe boundaries can a child successfully explore freedom, master tasks, and develop healthy initiative in their environment. The world is an unpredictable place, and we can flourish only if we can depend on someone stronger and wiser than ourselves to make it safe. We are creatures who are dependent on others for our well-being; it is something inscribed in the very fabric of our being and played out in the early growth and development of each and every one of us. We are contingent beings.

Contingency and Control

It will be worthwhile to sharpen this idea of contingency further. The dictionary defines it as something that depends on something else in order to happen. That something else, rather than certain, is a possibility, a chance, or an accidental occurrence. What makes us uncomfortable is the unpredictability of contingency and the need to depend on things we cannot fully control. But our hope for control will not be thwarted; even in the most common way we use the word, we restrain it, saying, "We've tried to imagine and provide for all possible contingencies." Yes, when we think of contingencies, we're thinking of how we can prepare for and negate each and every one of them.

But contingency goes deeper. It touches upon a question, a fear, perhaps an honest awareness if we are willing, that our existence is unnecessary, that we don't have to be here by any requirement that is written into the universe. As political scientist Glenn Tinder explains this more radical understanding of contingency, "To be contingent means that it is not one's essence to exist, nor, consequently, is it one's essence to be beautiful, wise, compassionate, or in any other way admirable. One's entire being, and one's every virtue, might not have been and may at any moment, cease to be."[2] But if we do not possess a reason within ourselves to be here, and if nothing in the makeup of the universe requires it, then if not by necessity, how am I here? Is it nothing but chance? Am I just an accident, randomly here? Or is there another possibility? Could my life be a gift, my existence a gracious given? And could there be a dependable parent, worthy of trust in the midst of life's uncertainties, who can help me explore my freedom within safe boundaries? If the biblical story at the beginning is true, that is exactly what our life is like.

The Original Plan

No one can call me a theologian in the formal sense of training and degrees, and I do not wish to act like one. But for many years I have desired to understand and analyze the practice and profession of medicine in the light of the biblical narrative. Here I have looked to make sense of our basic human nature, our susceptibility to sickness, and our capacity for healing, and it is here that I turn now, to the book of origins—Genesis—to try to understand our struggles for good health and good health care in our current society.

"In the beginning God created . . . ," and from these first words of the Bible proceeds the creation story for the next three chapters. Here we find the original plan, and it is surely good, as repeatedly in the first chapter everything God creates, from the sky to the earth, the moon to the stars, the vegetation to the creatures that depend on this vegetation for life and growth—each thing in its original form is called "good." The culmination of God's creation is us, the human being, a creature unique among all the creatures created before, because God creates for the first and only time "in his own image, in the image of God" (Gen. 1:27). We are *imago Dei*; yet, lest we forget our humble origins,[3] we are an image forged from the dust of the ground.

Looking at further events in the first two chapters of Genesis, we find that our struggle with contingency and control has roots in several essential elements of our basic human nature. First, we are created not because we must exist, to reiterate, but because God desires our existence; God is pleased to have created us. Emphasizing both gift and contingency, Catholic priest and philosopher Ivan Illich writes:

> What we discovered was a universe of continuous creation, lying continuously in the hands of God, a universe that would disappear if his hands disappeared, and which is necessary only insofar as it depends on his will. To contemplate such a universe was to cultivate a sense of contingency, a sense of having received as a free

gift one's own existence and the existence of everything which God has invented and brought forth.[4]

This view of ourselves, affirmed in the pages of Genesis, must be contemplated, Illich says, cultivated in order for us to begin and remain in right understanding of ourselves. We are not here by accident or by logical necessity but as a gift of a good God, whose intention for us is to grow and develop in a good and fruitful place.

A second element of our creation is that we are "breathing dust." In Genesis 2:7 we are told that God formed Adam from the "dust of the ground," making him a living being by "breath[ing] into his nostrils the breath of life"; the result, as Augustine described it, is *terra animata*, "animated earth."[5] This understanding of human nature is helpful in two ways. First, as a mixture of earthly dust and divine breath, we are "low" in our attachment to the earth, but also "high" in our attachment to God; it is somewhere between the "beasts and God" that we must try to find our place.[6] Second, the body and the soul are in intimate attachment; not two parts temporarily glued together but a union of spirit and flesh. German theologian Dietrich Bonhoeffer, in one of his early works, *Creation and Fall*, describes the essential unity:

> Man's body is not his prison, his shell, his exterior, but man himself. Man does not "have" a body; he does not "have" a soul; rather, he "is" body and soul. . . . The man who renounces his body renounces his existence before God the Creator.[7]

A third element of our nature is that we are created not independent but in dependence, both upon the earth and in relationship with one another and with God. We are placed in a garden but must till the land; this will produce the food upon which we will nourish our bodies that have come from this very same earth. God also knew from the beginning that "it is not good for the man to be alone" (Gen. 2:18). Dependent on intimate human relationship, Adam is given another like him, his wife, Eve, to help him and be his companion, as he will help her and be her companion. And then there is God, so close that they can hear the "sound of the LORD God as he was walking in the garden in the cool of the day" (Gen. 3:8).

The fourth element of our creation that helps as we consider contingency and control is provision; in the garden, the goodness of God provides all that is needed for human flourishing. There is good work to do, food that will grow from the cultivated ground that is good to the taste and good for the body, and companionship and mutual support in the relationship of man and woman, and they together with God.

As Genesis 2 ends, human creation lives in a good and safe place as contingent, dependent beings. Just like us, they have confronted the first developmental challenges of human existence and learned that they have a good and trustworthy heavenly parent. They are together in the garden "naked, and they felt no shame" (Gen. 2:25). But before them lies a new challenge, their next stage of development, the struggle between healthy autonomy or independence marked by shame and insecurity. They are about to face a decision, to continue to trust or demand their own way, to choose life or depend upon their own understanding. It is a choice for all the ages, one that presents itself in many forms today, as the following example illustrates.

A Present-Day Choice

One of the choices faced in medicine today is what to do when prenatal testing reveals that a baby has Down syndrome, a chromosomal abnormality that causes intellectual disability and developmental delays of varying severity. This testing is nearly always offered to pregnant women today, and while a few refuse it, most accept it. If the test reveals the presence of Down syndrome, families face the choice of whether to continue the pregnancy or abort the baby, since there is no option for treatment before birth. Most people,[8] in some studies over 85 percent,[9] choose the latter. The knowledge that their child will have Down syndrome, and, more importantly, the assumption that this will be bad, leads them to terminate the pregnancy. Rather than choosing the life of the child, they rely on their own understanding that the quality of this life will be bad.

Yet reality shows that their judgments mislead them. Surveys of parents, guardians, and siblings of children with Down syndrome reveal that a very high majority believe their lives are better and happier because these children are a part of their lives. When those with Down syndrome are asked, they report extremely high levels of satisfaction with their lives, much higher than when these surveys are done with an "unaffected" population.[10] Obviously, the knowledge we use to make our choices is not always reliable, though the choices we make may have life-and-death implications.[11]

A Tale of Two Trees: Life or Knowledge

Back in the garden, there were two trees. They were not out at the fringe; they stood right in the center: "In the middle of the garden were the tree of life and the tree of the knowledge of good and evil" (Gen. 2:9). As first introduced, the Tree of Life was simply there in place, available, with no evidence that Adam was forbidden to eat of it, because at this point in the story:

> Life was not problematic nor was it something to be pursued or seized. It was there, given, life in the presence of God. . . . Adam is not tempted to touch the tree of life, to lay violent hands on the divine tree in the middle; there is no need to forbid this; he would not understand the prohibition. He has life.[12]

Bonhoeffer goes on to explain that Adam's life, which he had no reason to grasp or possess, was only his through his unbroken relationship of trust and obedience with God. He had it in innocence, trusting God who had given it, and he had it in ignorance, not knowing the mechanics of it—only knowing that he had it. But he also had it in freedom, a freedom that could endanger his unbroken unity of trust and obedience.

Next to the Tree of Life, also in the middle, was the Tree of the Knowledge of Good and Evil. Though he was free to eat from any other tree in the garden, the fruit of this tree he was not to eat (Gen. 2:16–17). This tree introduced a prohibition to the freedom Adam had, a prohibition that shows something essential about our human nature:

> This man, who is addressed as one who is free, is shown his limit, that is to say, his creatureliness. In the prohibition Adam is ad-

dressed in his freedom and in his creatureliness, and by the prohibition his being is confirmed in its kind. It means nothing but
"Adam, thou art as thou art because of me, thy Creator; so be as
thou art. Thou art a free creature, so be a creature."[13]

To be as we are created means that as the tree stands in the middle
of the garden, so are our limits. Our limitations are not out at the edge
of our existence but at the center of our being. If our limits were at
the boundaries, we could always push them farther and farther out,
applying our reason and developing our technologies and solving the
problems that limit us at the edges of our lives. But that is not who we
are and how we have been made; our limits lie at the middle of our
creaturely existence and, if truth be told, we don't like that.

While much has been written and much can be said about what
happened next, suffice it to say Adam and Eve chose a world of their
own making rather than live in dependent creatureliness in the garden.
They, in this fundamental disunion with God, instead of knowing
only God who is good and knowing everything in God, chose to try
to become equal with God. As a result, we too, in deep disunion with
God, have come to understand ourselves as the origin of things and the
arbiter of good and evil, seeing ourselves as both creator and judge.
The core of the Serpent's temptation was to plant doubt that God
is good; for the first time they considered the contrary thought that
God, instead of being good and the giver of all good things, was with-
holding good things from them. Believing the lie, they reached out for
self-understanding and control and ate from the fruit of the Tree of the
Knowledge of Good and Evil. Nothing has been the same ever since.

There remains but one last thought to carry with us from these
first three chapters that has important implications for our pursuit of
health. It comes from the original meaning of the words "good and
evil" in Genesis 2:

> "Good and evil," *tob* and *ra*, here have a much wider meaning
> than the "good" and "evil" in our terminology. The words *tob*
> and *ra* speak of an ultimate division . . . which goes beyond moral
> discord, so that *tob* would perhaps also mean "full of pleasure"
> and *ra* "full of pain."[14]

Each of us, by virtue of our knowledge of *tob* and *ra*, assumes to know the difference between good and bad as the difference between right and wrong, in a moral or ethical sense. But in terms of the choices we make, there is another level of good and bad. We see good as that which is valuable, pleasant, and agreeable; knowing what will give us happiness, we can easily choose what we desire. Conversely, that which is unpleasant and causes pain, misery, and unhappiness we consider to be bad. In accord with the self-authorization that is a mark of our modern self, to know what is good and bad in this sense, and to determine our choices on that basis, has its origins "in the beginning."

But limiting ourselves to our possibilities and choosing among them based on our own understanding of good and bad are fraught with hazard. The faulty choices made by pregnant couples carrying a child with Down syndrome are but one example. Many decisions in life, especially health care decisions, must be made in anticipation of what will be, based on our assessment of the "good and bad" of anticipated outcomes. Highly influenced by the cultural air we breathe and our assumption that weakness and limitations are bad, we choose to control outcomes to exclude these possibilities whenever we can. In a world in which we fear what we cannot control, where contingencies must be reduced if not removed, our choices become restricted by our individual view of good and bad.

Life outside the Garden

Our personal judgments of good and bad carry a heavy weight in life beyond the garden. In the garden, like the child learning to exercise autonomy within limits, we exercised our freedom under protected conditions. In choosing to reject those limits for a life based on our own assessments, we lost something essential for healthy existence—a sense of place. In moving out into a limitless world, "even as this new world view affirmed a freedom of space it denied human existence its own proper place. While gaining infinite scope for movement man lost his own position in the realm of being."[15] In the garden, our human ancestors had a central place; outside it, we cease to experience a world that guarantees us a place in the total scheme of things. Not knowing where we belong, each one of us is forced to find our own way.

This places intense pressure on the reliability of our personal decisions, thus making us uniquely anxious in our choices. No wonder we plan incessantly in order to minimize chance and contingency. If we get it wrong, so we think, there is nothing in a hostile and impersonal universe that will rescue us. It certainly adds to the worry and anxiety with which most people pursue health and fear sickness today. Every uncertainty, every contingency that makes the world less predictable and more beyond our control, is a source of great dis-ease.[16] So we reach for every new technique and technology that will enable us to regain control. Alone and unsure of our place in an uncaring universe, we rely on our knowledge of good and bad and the technical solutions that promise deliverance.

Armed only with these resources, we struggle with a common problem in medicine today: how far to go. It comes up in numerous scenarios, from cancer treatment to testing for a potential problem. In each case, the most common fear is not going far enough, and this is fueled by the anxiety that something bad is out there, and if we stop too soon, "it" will happen. The related assumption, of course, is that in stopping too soon, we have lost the chance to control "it." One example, in an age of medical imaging that reveals the minutest details, is seeing something we weren't looking for while looking for something else. The problem is that we often don't know what to do about the fearful "it" we have found.

The patient, an elderly woman visiting her family for an extended stay from another country, had been experiencing pain in her leg for several months. One night the pain was unbearable, so her family took her to the emergency room. The treating physician, wanting to investigate if compression of a nerve in her back was causing the pain in her leg, ordered a CAT scan. The powerful images that looked inside her body revealed nothing unusual in her back but saw something in a completely different place. Though the findings, called "incidentalomas," were small and nonspecific, the word *abnormal* appeared on the report. In these situations, the fear of something bad may be generated by the doctor, the patient, or both. In this case, the medical system reacted with fear, which ultimately led to three additional studies and a painful biopsy before all were assured that this was nothing bad.

Besides the thousands of dollars spent to confirm "normal," one other casualty of "too much" in this case was the patient's actual concerns. In the pursuit of a normal test, the patient's ongoing pain was completely neglected. Her final reaction to high-tech medical care revealed her frustration: "I'm going back to my own country, where at least the doctors listen to the patient instead of looking at tests."

We can only be grateful for the powerful technology we have. Yet because the United States has more of it than any other country, we who have access to it are challenged to restrain our tendency to use it. But it will always be difficult to use wisely as long as the world is as bad as we fear. If only we could depend on something more than the power of our thinking and the tools we possess to stand between us and disaster.

Embracing Contingency

We are outside the garden now; we have eaten of the tree, and there is no going back. We know too much to return to its innocence and safety. The world is scary, accidental, and random, but the more we attempt to control the chaos, the more we fear what remains outside our control. Unfortunately, at one level the world of Genesis beyond chapter 3 confirms our fears. Outside the garden the human race faces a world of violence and pain; the soil is hard, the thorns are sharp, and from the moment Cain killed Abel, because Abel received a blessing that Cain did not, jealousy and envy have marked nearly every human story. Sarah envies Hagar, Jacob envies Esau, Laban envies Jacob, and Rachel envies Leah—over and over creating trouble, violence, and injustice.

The last third of Genesis is occupied by one final story, that of Joseph, whose envious older brothers sell him into slavery in Egypt. After selling Joseph, they assume they have solved their problem, but their view that having Joseph around was bad and selling him as a slave to Egypt was good created the problem of their father's grief, which was exceedingly bad. Though all his sons and daughters came to comfort him, "he refused to be comforted. 'No,' he said, 'I will continue to mourn until I join my son in the grave.' So his father wept for him" (Gen. 37:35). Jacob's sadness was slowly taking the life from him.

In the midst of unanticipated outcomes, failed attempts to make things better by our weak understanding of good and bad, and the ongoing presence of sickness and sadness, no matter what we do, we realize that despite our best efforts we truly do not know how it is going to be. It is hard to admit, but we are actors in a play who know only a small piece of the script, and we long for a director who knows what is next. As C. S. Lewis writes:

> We do not know the play. We do not even know whether we are in Act I or Act V. We do not know who are the major and who are the minor characters. The Author knows. . . . That it has a meaning we may be sure, but we cannot see it. When it is over, we may be told. We are led to expect that the Author will have something to say to each of us on the part that each of us has played. The playing it well is what matters infinitely.[17]

And "playing it well" we would gladly do, if only we knew we were a part of a story where contingent events do not bother the director, uncertainty and unpredictability do not disturb the plot, and surprise is even embraced as essential to the story.

After the garden, one might suppose God would leave us to our own devices; after all, if this is what humanity wanted, we got precisely what we reached for. But God does not stop caring, as the stories of the imperfect people of Genesis show over and over. And the book of Genesis does not end with Joseph's slavery or a father's grief.

The brothers have come to Egypt, where Joseph has risen to second in power under Pharaoh. And the father, reunited with his son, has died in peace. Now those who sold him into slavery stand before their powerful brother, afraid of the "bad" he will do in revenge for what they did to him. But Joseph has a different worldview. He believes that the universe is not random. He sees that personal knowledge of good and bad is not as reliable as we think. And he knows that the play has a director who is not disturbed by contingency, is completely in control of the script, and even absorbs and makes use of the mistakes of the actors. As the book of Genesis closes, Joseph's words to his brothers give us good news for an anxious age: "Don't be afraid. Am I in the place of God? You intended to harm me [plotted *ra* against me], but

God intended it for good [*tob*] to accomplish what is now being done, the saving of many lives. So then, don't be afraid" (Gen. 50:19–21).

That God remains an active agent in the world and is able to incorporate even the things we assume bad into a greater plan that can be good has the possibility to drastically change the way we pursue health and face sickness. Every time our health is in danger or we become ill, naturally and appropriately we will pursue the good of keeping or regaining our health. But are there times and places when other goods are possible? The idea that God is good, that God seeks communion with us, and that God has power and intention to work out good no matter the bad leaves us open to a much wider range of hopes and expectations than the singular one of health at all costs and with any technique.

But our ability to cultivate this sense of contingency and contemplate this vision of reality is constantly challenged by the prevailing worldview. We are trained in another way of seeing, that nothing of weakness, dependence, difficulty, pain, or suffering can ever have any meaning. It is to this way of seeing that we now turn.

What You See Depends

on How You Look

Disembodiment in Health Care, Part 1

The Clinical Gaze

The secret of the care of the patient is in caring for the patient.

Francis Peabody

In 1926 physician and teacher Francis Peabody presented a series of talks to Harvard medical students that reviewed the essentials of medical care in light of the new "scientific approach" that was exciting the world of academic medicine. His presentations revealed a growing concern that newly trained doctors would lose sight of the patient in the intense focus on the parts that science was learning to probe and understand:

> The most common criticism made at present by older practitioners is that young graduates have been taught a great deal about the mechanism of disease, but very little about the practice of

medicine—or, to put it bluntly, they are too "scientific" and do not know how to take care of patients.[1]

Admitting that some of this criticism by the older generation was nostalgic, if not an overidealization of their own training and experience, Peabody nevertheless realized that for a physician to properly care for a patient, such care demands a "whole relationship" of physician to patient. To see the patient properly, he said that the "clinical picture" is not just "a photograph of a sick man in bed; it [is] an impressionistic painting of the patient surrounded by his home, his work, his relations, his friends, his joys, sorrows, hopes and fears."[2]

Ending with his "secret" of patient care, reminding his generation that you cannot take care *of* a patient unless you actually and actively care *for* the patient, he believed this little lecture would be remembered long after any of his scientific writings had been forgotten. It remains one of the most cited and revered articles in medical literature.

Learning to See People in Parts

Most everyone who has had contact with modern medical education knows that it begins with the dissection of the human body in first-year anatomy class. The day they meet their cadaver is a defining moment for every medical student. Typically, the more uniquely human parts of the body such as the head and the hands are covered, unveiled only when the time comes to dissect them. Seeing them later, so the thinking goes, allows for *progressive desensitization*, which will make their eventual presentation less disturbing. Understanding the body in parts is an essential foundation for future doctors, who must learn to see people with a clinical eye if they are to make diagnoses out of symptoms and signs. But something must be surrendered on the way to gaining this view.

I recently asked some students in a first-year class to tell me about their reactions as the body was exposed over the nine-week period they completed anatomy. They described the need to see the body as separate from the soul, as an object that had lost its sacredness, and even as something inhuman as parts of the body were cut in half with a saw in order to show them in "sagittal section." This reordering of our view of the body is a difficult process. But in order to understand a thing analytically and then use this knowledge to alter and control it, we have to "suspend judgements of value about it, ignore its final cause (if any), and treat it in terms of quantity. This repression of elements in what would otherwise be our total reaction to it is sometimes very noticeable and even painful: something has to be overcome before we can cut up a dead man or a live animal in a dissecting room."[3]

Repressing our total reaction to the total person and an instinctive reverence for the human body is a process that begins in anatomy and is reinforced over and over in the course of medical school. I participate in a class called "Problem-Based Learning" for first-year and second-year medical students. Unabashedly, our intent is to teach them to think and speak as doctors. Based on the particular organ system being studied in the basic science curriculum, we take real patient cases and dissect them into problems, even using mnemonic devices to be sure no part of the body is neglected. As they grow in their ability to see what is wrong with the heart or the kidney, I fear they will lose their natural awareness that people are always more than the sum of their parts. These tensions will only increase as their training proceeds. In the third and fourth years they will join hospital teams as the most junior members, where the rush of patients needing care only increases the demand to see things in manageable packages. Shortcuts abound, and it is far easier to say, "Go see the liver in room 5," or, "Run down and assess the heart problem in the emergency room," than to say that Mrs. Smith, a retired schoolteacher who just lost her husband, is having chest pain and needs to be seen.

Graduating from medical school is an exhilarating experience, as we realize how far we have come and how much we have learned. But the experience is brief and possible only because of the mind's ability to forget what is coming—the most intense year of a physician's existence, the internship. I remember that year well. When I arrived at Boston City Hospital, the same institution where Francis Peabody worked until his death in 1927, I was appropriately excited and fearful, along with the thirty-four other new doctors who were joining me. But apart from the general concern that there would be no personal life outside medicine, something else worried me. I feared that my training was draining away an important piece of me. I knew I needed to continue to grow in the clinical gaze, seeing patients as a set of problems, thinking in terms of parts, and understanding dysfunction in order to restore function so that the practice of medicine, and I as its practitioner, could do its job. But was I losing the ability to see the patient as a person?

One patient stands out from those distant days. He was a homeless man admitted to the hospital for abdominal pain and breathing trouble. Initial studies showed a number of potential problems, so a series of specialists was called to consult, all seeing him through their own particular lens. The nephrologists wanted a number of kidney tests. The gastroenterologists said the patient needed a liver biopsy but also an upper intestinal endoscopy to check for bleeding. Then the radiologist called to say his initial X-rays were abnormal, and he would need further imaging with contrast to enhance the picture—but only if the patient's kidneys could withstand the potential dangers of the dye. Finally, the pulmonologists said the patient needed a bronchoscopy, but only if the gastroenterologists said his liver was strong enough for anesthesia.

Over several days, as we worked to get everything done without one domino knocking over another, I learned that the patient had become homeless after losing his job and then drinking too much to numb the pain. His drinking damaged his relationships with family, and when his wife told him she wanted a divorce, he became more depressed and drank more heavily. In the month leading up to his admittance, he had begun vomiting, even seeing blood once or twice, but he didn't know where to go because he had no insurance. One day he was having so much pain that he could barely breathe, so the shelter where he was staying called an ambulance, which brought him to the emergency room where I first met him.

After three weeks in the hospital, with all the tests negative and his symptoms improved, it was time to send him home, even though he did not have a home. When I told my supervisor that I wanted to talk to someone who could help him find a job, he told me that was not our problem. Though it was true that we had carried out our responsibilities correctly, I knew we hadn't addressed our patient's real need. I figured it wouldn't be long before I saw him again if he returned to the streets and started drinking again. As many in my profession desire, and as my predecessor Francis Peabody had recommended, I wanted to care for the whole patient. But the pressures of becoming a good doctor can frequently push aside our best intentions.

The Story of the Stethoscope

Seeing people in parts in order to understand their problems is closely related to another chapter in the manual of medical training, the need to develop professional distance. At the same time that we dig deep into the body to understand its workings and make diagnoses, we are taught to step back personally so that we can dispassionately determine what our patient needs. At one level, we protect ourselves against emotional burnout by staying detached from our patient's lives, which can, at times, be quite tragic. But more logically, we are told that this "experience-far" view,[4] exalting "disengaged reason as the royal road to knowledge,"[5] enables us to remain unbiased and objective in our perspective. The knowledge we obtain by this means is "studied quite independent of us, where we don't need to understand it at all through our involvement with it, or the meanings it has in our lives."[6]

Applied to medicine, we step back from too much awareness of, or involvement in, people's individual lives so that we will not impede the formation of an objective clinical gaze. So we start by listening to what patients tell us, but not too much or for too long, because their report of what is going on, their symptoms, is subjective and fraught with bias; what we seek are objective signs. At first we gained these unbiased signs through a careful reading of the body by a thorough physical exam, a hands-on approach of direct palpation and probing. But before too long, we introduced our first technology for better information. It is the story of the first stethoscope, which has been the iconic image of medicine ever since.

It was September 13, 1816, and Rene Laënnec, perhaps the greatest physician of the early nineteenth century, was examining a woman with symptoms of a diseased heart at the Necker Hospital in Paris.[7] His efforts to examine the patient by the usual methods of "percussion and application of the hand were of little avail on account of the great degree of fatness."[8] The other method of examination, the application of the ear to the front of the chest, was "rendered inadmissible by the age and sex of the patient."[9] In the wink of an eye, the world of clinical medicine was completely transformed when Laënnec, remembering some principles of acoustics, rolled up a sheaf of paper into a cylinder, placed one end on his patient's chest and put his ear to the other. For the first time he heard the augmented sounds of a heartbeat transmitted along the length of the tube, and the stethoscope was born.

This basic but helpful technique for better examination initially created but a foot of space between doctor and patient. But ever since this first separation, we have been moving farther and farther away in the search for more objective information. Ever-evolving techniques produce sharper images and more precise test results but at increasing distance from the patient. Once, we surrounded the bed of the patient to discuss the case; now we conference around computer screens, looking at images, evaluating numbers, and managing the function of each and every organ without ever having to see the patient. We don't even have to see the patient to listen to the heartbeat anymore; a digital stethoscope can capture those audio waveforms and transmit them to our phone, tablet, or computer. With each step away we gain a deeper sense that our experience-far view is steeped in objectivity for the benefit of the patient. But the farther away we get, the more likely we see the body as separate from the person, ultimately a profound partition that views the body as "it," an infinitely malleable and ever-changing product of our own perspective and pursuits.

Managing bodies apart from souls takes on a particular tone in our day because of the power of our technology. But it is only a rewrite of an old theme, which is worth looking at if only to accentuate the unique dangers of this most recent iteration.

An Ancient Heresy Revisited

The idea that the body can be treated apart from the soul is a basic and ever-recurring misunderstanding. A very specific form called "Gnosticism" emerged as a movement in the first two centuries of the Christian era. Looking at the natural world, most specifically the body, as a hindrance to the soul, it emphasized escape from the body through a secret and special knowledge of the divine.[10] Early Gnosticism even went so far as to view the created order as a mistake, as pastor and author Philip Lee points out, in direct opposition to a good creation that was the prevailing Jewish and Christian view:

> The material world itself is the result of a cosmic faux pas. . . . The ancient gnostic, looking at the world through despairing eyes, saw matter in terms of decay, place in terms of limitation, time in terms of death. In light of this tragic vision, the logical conclusion seemed to be that the cosmos itself—matter, place, time, change, body, and everything seen, heard, touched or smelled—must have been a colossal error. [11]

In searching for a "gnostic type" that would link gnostics of all times, Lee proposes a particular mood, one of despair with current reality.[12] Since our current view of the body is at root a despairing one, it is not surprising that the way we look at the body with the clinical gaze incorporates many elements of this gnostic typology. What heavily updates the new version of this old dualism is the technological progress that defines today's medical encounter with the body. Wendell Berry clarifies the change:

> For many centuries there have been people who looked upon the body, as upon the natural world, as an encumbrance of the soul, and so have hated the body, as they have hated the natural world, and longed to be free of it. They have seen the body as intolerably imperfect by spiritual standards. More recently, since the beginning of the technological revolution, more and more people have looked upon the body, along with the rest of the natural creation, as intolerably imperfect by mechanical standards. They see the body as an encumbrance of the mind . . . and so they hate it and long to be free of it.[13]

The body as machine, functioning for better or worse on the basis of the quality of its working parts, becomes the acting metaphor for a medical gnosticism that, much like ancient Gnosticism, offers a form of salvation that will free us from the limits of the body, but now by way of the special knowledge of science. The following example, though extreme, is utterly consistent with this view of the body.

In a real scenario, an infertile couple decided to solve their problem piece by piece. Making good use of the Internet, they chose sperm from an athletic man with a 4.0 grade-point average and picked a premed student to donate the eggs. Then they placed an order for a gestational carrier, providing a "rentable" uterus for temporary housing. After finding a fertility clinic that would put the pieces together and paying all the fees, they ultimately came home with their purchase, and a good deal at that, since they had twins. But their happiness was short-lived. The surrogate mother, when she discovered there was mental illness in the adoptive family, sought a court order to reclaim the children. With none of the individuals involved having any genetic relationship to the children, it has created a conundrum for the legal system and raised significant ethical questions.[14]

Even if we open a Pandora's box of legal and moral complications, to escape the body we will willingly bow at the feet of modern biomedicine as the possessor of special knowledge and techniques. Let's consider the implications of medical gnosticism for a more common reality: the control of pain.

The Measurement and Eradication of Pain

A body in pain has confused and challenged the human experience since the beginning of time. But what if, refuting all prior history of pain as a multifaceted and complex bodily experience with diffuse and multiple causes, it is just a bunch of nerve endings transmitting aversive signals to the brain? That's something we can quantify, medicate, and eradicate.

So we made pain a disease, not a symptom,[15] because diseases can be categorized, not just experienced. Once defined by a diagnosis, the medical community took responsibility for its cure. With the power of the clinical gaze, we measured it on a scale of one to ten, climbed an increasingly potent ladder of pain medications to alleviate it, and ended up with many patients on multiple strong pain medications for a very long time.

The beginning of the use of chronic narcotics for noncancer pain can be traced to a report in 1986 showing safe use in a small series of cases.[16] Though most states continued to prohibit their use in non-cancer pain for longer than three months, by the late 1990s these laws were dramatically loosened. From 1999 to 2014, sales of prescription narcotics in the United States quadrupled.[17] During this same time frame, overdose deaths from prescription narcotics also quadrupled, surpassing deaths from heroin and cocaine combined.[18] Drug overdose deaths, driven primarily by the increase in deaths caused by prescription narcotics and the increased use of heroin by those addicted to prescription narcotics,[19] has now overtaken motor vehicle crashes as the leading cause of injury death in the United States,[20] producing a public health emergency. A reevaluation of these powerful medicines for pain has led to a rapid reversal in many of the aggressive recommendations for its treatment in the face of this epidemic of misuse and death.[21]

We started with a well-founded desire to reduce pain. We assumed pain to be primarily the result of chemicals provoking certain parts of the nervous system to fire excessively, on the gnostic belief that it is a merely mechanical function and fully controllable. But along the way of treating pain as a solvable problem, we ended up with a generation of individuals addicted to prescription pain medications.

So a simple biomedical approach to complex realities such as pain created a national problem. Clearly a clinical gaze that reduces the body to the physiological function of its parts is too small a view. So why not enlarge the gaze?

Extending the Clinical Gaze

The development of the reductive clinical gaze began over two hundred years ago, when the science of medicine first began to see the living body from the perspective of the dead body dissected into parts.[22] This gaze has given its practitioners great power to separate and analyze for the purpose of fixing or improving. But in the last forty years, acknowledging its limitations, the gaze has been extended into a new model of patient engagement, the biopsychosocial approach, with another layer added more recently, giving us biopsychosocial-spiritual medicine.

This enlargement of the gaze at first blush seems a good and wise response to an overly reductive biomedical view. By adding these aspects of the person to the clinical gaze, this new model allows a greater opportunity to see the whole person. Considering pain, now we can incorporate how people experience it, the societal and cultural context that influences their experience of it, and even if their religious perspective helps them find meaning in it. With this more holistic view of patients, we will be more inclined to draw close and see them as unique persons instead of standing back looking at their parts.

But what first appears as a larger view bears closer examination, if only because the clinical gaze is never a neutral observer. Wherever the gaze is directed, because its purpose is to fix or improve, everything it sees must submit to analysis and categorization to achieve that end. When turned toward psychological processes, family dynamics, or religious behaviors, "scientifically rational approach[es] to behavioral and psychosocial data"[23] are expected to produce measurable improvements.

Physician and ethicist Jeffrey Bishop, who has followed the development of the medical model in his carefully argued book *The Anticipatory Corpse*,[24] shows the outcome of this endeavor for the process of grief. First we form a model with stages and time frames. Then we create assessment tools to measure a patient's grieving process according to the model. With lines drawn between acceptable and unacceptable grief, we promote activities to fix any problems, after which we reassess and obtain new numbers. Undeterred by the idiosyncrasies of grieving, the patient is better if the measurements have improved. With unrelenting demand for efficiency and effectiveness, even God should show value when stared at by the clinical gaze; or to put it more scientifically, spiritual attachments must be measured along the continuum of improvement if the patient's religious practice is to be validated.

Unfortunately, extending the gaze has not in and of itself brought us closer to the particularities of individual patients. Despite its admirable inclusion of more of the patient, the demand of the gaze for calculation and control keeps us at a distance and the patient in parts. Rather than walking with patients on their unique path, we remain back so that we can measure grief. The only thing left is to collect the data and report it in the digital world, where a favorable "composite performance score" will assure us we have effectively and efficiently cared for our patients.

The Clinical Gaze in Electronic Mode

The electronic health record may yet be the most powerful change in how we see patients in the twenty-first century. The interpretation of a patient through a screen is nothing new, having exerted its influence decades ago with the broad use of computers. Many a patient has already been seen primarily through the laboratory results or medical images brought to us on a screen in the nurses' station or the doctor's office.

But since the screen entered the exam room, everything must bow to its power. Now the parts of the patient must fit its electronic categories—only diminishing the patient further by forcing them into fixed templates of auto-populated fields that help us do our work. And the data it reports and the standards it expects are always with us, filling the room with numbers that tell us what we need to do, regardless of how context-poor and fictional the account they give.

Then on October 1, 2015, already looking at the screen more and the patient less, suddenly the room shakes. An explosion in coding precision has just transformed the thirteen thousand possible diagnoses in the old medical billing code into sixty-eight thousand possible diagnoses in a new one.[25] Never before has a patient been broken into this many parts, with the pieces so predetermined, and the categories so tight. Welcome to the age of the electronic clinical gaze.

Some Patients Refuse to Fit

No matter how hard we try, some people won't be reduced to parts and cannot be placed in any fixed category. One patient always comes in with his wife, who makes jokes at his expense that make him, and you, laugh. He always asks how you are before you have a chance to ask how he is. He gives you a coffee cup with your name on it because he thinks you have done so much for him. He always takes his medicine, never misses an appointment, is stoic when in pain, happy in health, and always appreciative no matter what you do. You look forward to seeing him, and whenever he comes, you always end up turning from the screen so you can talk to him. You cannot help but see him as a person with a past that interests you, a present you enjoy being a part of, and a future you hope you can help make better.

Another patient misses appointments frequently and forgets to take his medicines for no obvious reason. Then he comes without an appointment and wants to be seen right away because it is urgent. Sometimes he comes in drunk and angry but two days later calls to say how sorry he is for the way he behaved. You think about him a lot. He's only fifty, but his kidneys are failing and he will soon need dialysis unless you can get him to take his medicines. No matter how much you try, you can't make him fit into the template of the electronic medical record—so you finally give up, turn from the screen, and listen to the patient. He tells you about a son who won't talk to him anymore, then he starts crying and thanks you for listening. He says he'll take his medicine from now on, and you say that's good, even though you know it probably won't happen. You cannot help but see him as a person, with a past that is bad, a present that is sad, and a future you wish you could make better, though you probably won't.

Patients who refuse to fit give hope that the individuality of patients, always at risk before a clinical gaze that must prove its mettle in measurable outcomes, will still have a place in the future of health care. But losing the individual in the rules and regulations of parts that fit in the boxes of an electronic record is only one side of the disembodied gaze of medical science. In the next chapter we will step back further, looking at the patient as an "average" one of many, thereby making sure that our experience-far view is unassailably neutral and objective.

5

Disembodiment in Health Care, Part 2

The Statistical Gaze

In statistical affairs . . . the first care before all else is to lose sight of the man taken in isolation in order to consider him only as a fraction of the species. It is necessary to strip him of his individuality to arrive at the elimination of all accidental effects that individuality can introduce into the question.[1]

In 1980 I was a third-year medical student on a pediatric rotation in New York City. The hospital was part of the Columbia Presbyterian Medical Center, located on the Upper West Side of Manhattan very near to where New Jersey traffic pours into the city via the George Washington Bridge. One of the cars that traversed the bridge that year brought a mother and a father to the hospital with their sick child. Soon after being admitted, the child was diagnosed with leukemia.

One night I was in the room finishing my rounds, and the father began to talk. He was beside himself with guilt, sure that it was his fault his son had cancer—all because he chose to live in northern New Jersey. He had recently heard about a study with statistical evidence linking EMF (electric and magnetic fields) from power lines to cancer, particularly leukemia and brain cancer in children. He had moved his family to New Jersey five years ago, had chosen to buy a house under a number of power lines, and now his son had leukemia. It seemed an inadequate hypothesis to explain why his son had cancer. But for him the statistics were proof, making sense out of the non-sense of a child with cancer, even if they proved his guilt. Though I had spent the first twenty years of my life in northern New Jersey, I never thought of it as a cancer risk. But then I never had to try to understand a world where my two-year-old son had leukemia.

The idea that living close to power lines could cause leukemia was first suggested by a study done in 1979. Further evidence continued to support the link, leading to research in 1988 that became one of the more commonly cited studies connecting EMF with childhood cancer. But later analysis of the results and methodology revealed a pronounced bias. It turns out their method of choosing a control group, a common technique called "random digital dialing," produced an unfair comparison for the study group. In fact, the data showed that the risk of leukemia and brain cancer rises not just with exposure to EMF but also with higher levels of breast-feeding, maternal smoking, and traffic density.[2] Rather than supporting the hypothesis that EMF causes childhood cancer, the scatter of random associations suggested the real causative factors were still missing.

Yet public concern continued, leading Congress to authorize further investigations in the 1990s. These showed no consistent, significant link between cancer and power line EMFs. A 1999 report by the National Institute of Environmental Health Sciences (NIEHS) concluded, "The scientific evidence suggesting that ELF-EMF exposures pose any health risk is weak."[3] But it goes on to state, "The NIEHS concludes that ELF-EMF exposures cannot be recognized as entirely safe because of weak scientific evidence that exposure may pose a leukemia hazard." In essence, science is unable to prove a negative, including whether low-level EMFs are completely risk free.[4] Thus the question persists and will continue, with the newest concern focusing on the exposure to EMF from cell phones.[5]

Increasingly, medical science is approving only one source of knowledge, that which is "proven" by statistics. If something is cloaked in numbers, it must be true. But incomplete data, multiple sources of bias, and bewildering complexity producing results of implausible precision are making it difficult to determine when the results are valid and, more importantly, when the outcomes are meaningful for our individual lives. With each new study, the reportedly true and possibly dangerous is moving farther and farther away from anyone's own real-life experience. How did statistical evidence grow to become such an unquestioned authority in our current world?

The Development of the Statistical View

Bloodletting, a remedy with a three-thousand-year history, was never so widely employed as it was in France between 1815 and 1835, due primarily to the influential teaching of the charismatic physician Francois-Joseph-Victor Broussais. An enthusiastic supporter of the "irritation" model of disease, he taught that bleeding the patient was a remedy for many conditions, including "moderate inflammations of the encephalon" and "violent sanguineous congestions of the brain."[6] Many denounced these methods, particularly those in rural communities, claiming that the "pitiless leeches . . . quickly exhaust the blood that remains in their veins" and "has made more blood flow than the most pitiless conqueror."[7]

But rural opposition was no match for the urban prestige of Broussais and the power of his medical model. No one could dispute the science of the great doctor—until 1835, when Pierre Charles Alexandre Louis published a series of statistical evaluations of bloodletting that showed it was totally ineffective.[8] For the first time in medicine the "numerical method" of large groups stood up and proved its worth, showing it could debunk unfounded theory with a new form of evidence.

Philosopher and historian of science Ian Hacking sees the years surrounding Louis's publication, more specifically the nineteenth century, as a turning point. It was during this time, he writes, that "society became statistical. A new type of law came into being, analogous to the laws of nature, but pertaining to people. The new laws were expressed in terms of probability. They carried with them the connotations of normalcy and of deviations from the norm."[9] Hacking goes on to describe the increasing infiltration of statistical analysis in medicine, politics, and society, initially taking place in England and France, but rapidly spreading throughout Europe and into the New World. From investigating the rate of death, the ratio of male to female births, the question of whether Parisians or Londoners were more suicidal, or why certain sicknesses occurred more in winter than summer, it was the laws of large numbers, central tendencies, and bell-shaped distribution curves that proved invaluable for predicting behaviors, determining likelihoods, and directing decisions. A few voices in this period protested an overdependence on numbers and calculations to define reality, from sources as disparate as Neitzsche to Dostoyevsky. But for the most part, its detractors were no match for the evolving power of the method, and a statistical view of the world bounded into the twentieth century with growing confidence and vigor.

The field of numerical statistics has exploded since that time. In medicine, the importance of statistics, initially marginalized to public health and epidemiology, has slowly extended its territory to decision making about individual patients. The widespread use of statistical medicine in clinical settings broke through with the publication of the Evidence-Based Medicine Working Group in 1992.[10] Today every medical school has expanded its training in biostatistics as a basic necessity for evaluating a medical literature so heavily dependent on statistical confidence limits, odds ratios, and relative and absolute risk reductions to confirm its value.

But underneath this growing cauldron of statistics and probabilities that have redefined the practice of medicine in the twenty-first century lies a fundamental contradiction: the evidence of evidence-based medicine (EBM) is derived from groups, whereas medicine is applied to individuals. Just as the prophets of the past warned us,[11] the ever-present danger is that we will lose the individual in the numbing rush of numbers and calculations. In this chapter we will focus on three ways that today's statistical gaze can forget persons: when we have a disease, when we have an aberration, and when we have a risk.

When We Have a Disease

Whenever we are sick, one of our fundamental concerns is what will happen next. Will we recover? Will we get worse? Could we die? As far back as Hippocrates, the ability to predict the outcome of illness, to prognosticate, has always been considered one of the most important marks of a good physician:

> It appears to me a most excellent thing for the physician to culti-vate Prognosis; for by foreseeing and foretelling, in the presence of the sick, the present, the past, and the future . . . he will be the more readily believed to be acquainted with the circumstances of the sick; so that men will have confidence to intrust themselves to such a physician. And he will manage the cure best who has fore-seen what is to happen from the present state of matters.[12]

Hippocrates then proceeds to instruct the young physician in the skills of prognostication. One should observe the countenance of the patient in acute disease, he counsels. If reclining on either the right or left side with the whole body in a relaxed state, this is a good sign, while a pinched nose, hollow eyes, and collapsed temples is a worri-some portent. Even the movement of the hands is considered impor-tant to the observant physician, for "when in acute fevers, pneumonia, phenitis, or headache, the hands are waved before the face, hunting through empty space, as if gathering bits of straw, picking the nap from the coverlet, or tearing chaff from the well—all such symptoms are bad and deadly."[13]

Today, we still prognosticate but with a much different approach, less likely to observe the patient and far more inclined to look at survival statistics or disease progression likelihoods. In one sense this is more accurate. Having data to show what has happened to people with disease X, we can calculate the average survival and how existing treatments alter that outcome. Patients currently with disease X can look at these numbers as a way to predict what will happen to them. But what do they see? And can they find what they are looking for?

Some will doubt the validity of the data. A few will admire the importance of this knowledge for advancing the practice of medicine. Many will be overwhelmed by the sheer quantity of information, while others find it helpful to know that 40 percent of people treated with treatment Y will survive for five years. But none of them will find the answer they are most looking for: "Will I survive?" Because whatever the statistics show, no one is just an average.

Stephen Gould, a well-known biologist and historian of science, died in 2002. What was important about the date of his death is that it was twenty years after being diagnosed with mesothelioma, a cancer that had a median survival of eight months. Shortly after his diagnosis, he used his understanding of statistics to write a personal story, "The Median Isn't the Message."[14] Gould saw in the statistical picture of his disease two major elements: the central tendency, which gave him a median survival of eight months, and the variation around this central tendency, which was more skewed to the right, meaning some people had a chance of living for many years with his disease. His scientific prowess enabled him to understand that the median, which would lead most people to conclude, "I will probably be dead in eight months," was the abstraction, and the variation around this central average was the deeper reality of life. As he saw it, "variation is nature's only irreducible essence. Variation is the hard reality, not a set of imperfect measures of central tendency."[15]

Certainly, statistical distributions of outcomes for patients similar to us can help us to consider our options and make our decisions. But deep down we know we are more than an abstraction. "It occurred to me that my relationship with statistics changed as soon as I became one," one doctor wrote when diagnosed with metastatic lung cancer at age thirty-six. "The angst of facing mortality has no remedy in probability."[16] For each one, there is no percentage or probability—either we will get better or get worse, improve with treatment or not, be alive in eight months or in five years or not. No number, no matter how high, should have the power to convince us we have won; nor should any number, no matter how low, stop us from living our lives with all the vigor we have for as long as we have it.

When We Have an Aberration

The use of the "normal" in medical contexts has usually depended on seeing deviation to either side as disease. It comes from an old idea that health is a balance between excess and deficiency. A typical example is vitamins—too little Vitamin A causes blindness, too much Vitamin A is toxic to bone and skin, and in between is a normal, healthy amount. Framed within a general idea of balance, and when applied to numerous physiologic mechanisms, the idea is sound. But its extension to the wider context of human behavior has produced a profound change in the way we use medicine. In a process called "medicalization," many characteristics previously acceptable within a normal distribution become pathologic aberrations, making "the benign and sterile-sounding word 'normal' . . . one of the most powerful ideological tools of the twentieth century."[17]

With variations on the theme, the simplest definition of medicalization is when previously nonmedical problems become defined (and ultimately treated) as medical problems. This process can be beneficial. Childbirth, for example, has historically been a nonmedical experience and still is for many. Yet the use of the medical principles of hygiene and sterility has prevented numerous infections at this crucial moment of life, showing how a judicious application of medicalization to a common condition can produce broad benefit. Beyond narrow examples like this, however, the world becomes much more complicated. As we consider two examples of overmedicalization, we are not looking for the elusive line between normal and abnormal but for how medicalization affects our gaze.

Depression in adults has been characterized and categorized with increasing specificity over the last thirty years. In *The Loss of Sadness: How Psychiatry Transformed Normal Sorrow into Depressive Disorder*[18] authors Horwitz and Wakefield describe a watershed change, strongly advanced in 1980 through the publication of the third edition of the *Diagnostic and Statistical Manual of Mental Disorders* (DSM), that classified mental problems according to a set of symptoms, regardless of cause. Though the criteria for diagnosis allowed comparisons across institutions and research programs, it too easily labeled patients "depressed" in the absence of context. "Medicalizing" sadness and melancholy has dramatically increased the number of people diagnosed with depression and produced a proliferation of pharmaceutical products that treat it.[19] Though definitions continue to evolve, and many people still do not receive adequate care for this important condition, the fact that over 10 percent of Americans over age twelve take an antidepressant medication daily suggests a powerful medicalization effect.[20]

Like depression, ADHD (Attention Deficit and Hyperactivity Disorder) in children lacks a physiologic test to prove its presence; therefore the diagnosis depends heavily upon human judgment and cultural context. In the United States, with broader definitions and wider awareness of the medications available to treat it, the number of children diagnosed has dramatically increased, making over one in ten children "sick" with this disorder.[21] Some of this increase may represent better detection. But the size of the change and the labeling of so many children as patients needing potentially toxic treatment have changed our view of childhood in general, and acceptable behavior in children more specifically.

Labeling 10 percent of the population diseased, whether with depression, ADHD, or any other condition, creates a widening of medical jurisdiction, authority, and practice into everyday life. Medicine grows in power to define what is normal, whether it be behavior, body shape, or ability. The number of people taking daily medication skyrockets, with greater risk of side effects from the treatment used to solve the medicalized problem. All of this explodes the need for professional care, whether to prescribe pills, offer therapy, or deal with the side effects of treatment.

Most importantly, it changes how we see ourselves and others. Much of human difference is no longer absorbed within a broader social context but stands apart as undesirable and stigmitizable characteristics of the individual. Individuals struggle to fit or belong based on the new categories of normal and abnormal. The label of "abnormal" or "diseased" changes self-perception, with new identities formed that are heavily defined by the medical diagnosis. Some take the diagnosis fatalistically, assuming the role of the "sick" patient, which can hinder social and personal development and have lifelong consequences.

One patient, on being told she had social anxiety disorder, accepted the diagnosis as a permanent limitation and gave up trying to function in the world. Never seeking employment or pursuing school or relationship opportunities, her diagnosis doomed her to a disabled and restricted life.

Despite its negative effects, medicalization is proving to be a durable social phenomenon capable of evolving in response to changing attitudes. For example, people today often reject "conforming to a norm" as an archaic idea, as many observant readers are aware, with greater emphasis on finding one's own way. Keeping basic principles intact, medicalization has adapted to this movement of late modernity by morphing into "customization."[22] The next tattoo, body piercing, body sculpting, or health product chosen looks like a personal choice. But rather than a rejection of norms, customization accepts a multiplicity of norms, with a smaller reference group to inform the standard. With the growing capability of technology and widening access to its power, more and more people can alter their body or the way they feel according to this broader definition of norms. Bodily life continues as adjustable only with more variety—actually more flexible, reconfigurable, and transformable—than ever before, and still heavily dependent on medicalized solutions to achieve the more individual norm.[23]

When We Have a Risk

One of the greatest ways statistical thinking disembodies our gaze is in the transformation of our view of risk of disease. Here we learn to experience the smallest of likelihoods with the greatest of fears through the power of numbered probabilities. Whether it is a risk of exposure, as in the case of EMF, or a risk tied to age, test result, family history, or cholesterol level, we come to define our present in the shadow of what might happen in a distant future. What really matters today gets pushed aside by future worries, a deceptive and distracting enterprise,[24] as the following case illustrates.

Mr. Smith was a regular patient, but he came only once or twice a year. More like a check-in than a checkup, he usually restricted the conversation to the few things he needed to check off so that he could go on with life, confident that all was well. His last visit was particularly exasperating to his primary care practitioner.

Physician: How are you today?

Patient: Fine, Doc.

Physician: Any changes since your last visit?

Patient: No, everything is the same.

Physician: Last time we talked about my concern that drinking more than twelve beers and smoking two packs of cigarettes a day were beginning to affect your health. Have you thought any more about that?

Patient: I've been doing this all my life, Doc. Like I told you before, I feel fine.

Physician: I continue to be concerned with your use of cigarettes and alcohol. Your blood pressure is higher today and . . .

Patient: Oh, don't worry, it's probably stress. I'm going on a little vacation, and that should help. I'm taking a trip to Southeast Asia. Do I need any malaria pills or shots?

Physician: I can look into that. But I think we're missing the . . .

Patient: Sorry to interrupt, Doc, but what I'm really worried about is my prostate. I don't want to get cancer. I've heard about the PSA test.[25] Can we do that?[26]

Though the physician knows his worry about prostate cancer is sidelining the more important discussion about his present habits and choices, she cannot escape her responsibility to address his concern. Caught in the abstraction of the present by the patient's perceived risk of future cancer, she attempts to explain the risks and benefits of the screening test. It won't be easy to help him understand that though it does detect cancer that would otherwise be missed, most of the cancer discovered will be slow-growing and have no impact on his future life; in addition, if he is diagnosed with cancer and chooses treatment, it is more likely that he will have side effects from the treatment than that the treatment will save him from dying of prostate cancer.[27]

Despite her best efforts to keep it simple but accurate so he can make an informed decision, as often happens, by the end of her explanation his eyes have glazed over. In the end he has the PSA test, not because he understands the pros and cons but because it is the test to do if you want to know you don't have prostate cancer. (Unfortunately, she didn't have time to explain the false-negative rate, that is, the frequency with which the test is normal but the patient nevertheless has prostate cancer.) Comforted by the normal result, he heads off to Southeast Asia, leaving his most important risks for future health unaddressed, believing all is well because he's seen his doctor and his number is good.

Much danger lies in an overdependence on a probabilistic interpretation of our lives. Though the gaze of risk awareness displaces the embodied present with a disembodied future, we accept being an abstract average member of a statistically analyzed population if it will enlarge our sense of safety. In an "oncophobic" society that fears cancer as synonymous with death, the PSA example shows how well current programs to reduce cancer risk fit this approach. Taking a test and getting a "normal" result reduces our sense of vulnerability. Little does it matter that many of our efforts show little likelihood of benefit or sometimes produce more harm than good;[28] if the right numbers are attached, we accept these disembodied probabilities as objective knowledge to maintain the illusion that life is still safe. Even if we might neglect more important choices in our immediate life, as our patient does, or let recurrent worry about the future inhibit our present health, as often happens, we do so anyway in the name of control. But there is another way to use probability and statistics.

At the end of the day, this doctor has one more patient. He comes every three months to check his blood pressure, which is usually good because he takes his medicine every day. Today he wants to know if he should be taking a pill to lower his cholesterol. Using an online program based on age, cholesterol level, and blood pressure, she tells him that four out of a hundred people like him are predicted to have a heart attack over the next ten years. On the other hand, if all one hundred people take a daily cholesterol-lowering medication for ten years, only three people will have a heart attack.[29] "You mean only one person will be saved from a heart attack, and for the other ninety-nine it makes no difference?" he asks. She is pleased he understands. Finally, after telling him that the medication causes side effects in seven out of a hundred people, he makes his decision. "I'm not going to do it. It's too little benefit for all that medicine, with a greater chance of problems. Anyway, nothing's sure in life. I'll just keep taking my blood pressure medicine, exercise, and avoid smoking. I think that's the best I can do."

Clearly, both the patient and the medical profession can be guilty of misusing probabilities to control an unknown future. But when both are aligned toward the value that probabilities can have for informing present decisions and encouraging healthy behavior, the result can be satisfying for patient and practitioner.

Lost in (Statistical) Space

The mythical power of numbering, which lies at the core of scientific reasoning, has always promised to give an account of the world without changing it. At its highest point, we "rise above and beyond our particular, narrow biased view of things, to a view from everywhere" and become the impartial spectator.[30] In prior days we used this universal view of natural science to focus on small problems, investigate the mechanisms of specific diseases, and discover strongly determinative cause-and-effect relationships. But in an age of healthier populations, at least in economically advanced countries, we are driven more and more to medicalize normal events, turn risks into diseases, and make the unknown of individual disease outcomes into predictable events. Ignoring the limitations, probability and statistics have become our most useful allies in this project. Forcing them to function beyond their ability to show meaningful associations, they have become for us impartial law producing unassailable truth.

But "the paradox of the triumph of science and technology is that to the degree that a person perceives himself as an example of, a specimen of, this or that type of social creature or biological genotype, to precisely this same degree does he come short of being himself."[31] Seen as law-abiding members of a population that obeys statistical rules of risk, or disease outcome, or normality, we become less of who we are and more of what the numbers tell us we are, should be, or might become. As science progresses along this line, even as it benefits us in general, it distances itself farther and farther from real people in real time while making us more fearful of unlikely possibilities lying far in the future.

The people whom Gulliver found on the island of Laputa, as we've already seen, were advanced in science but overly fearful of improbable future events. Curiously, they also found it difficult to stay connected to the concrete realities of present life. When Gulliver toured their land, he noticed their buildings were poorly constructed; because geometry was far too practical for their enlightened minds, there wasn't a single right angle in any of the rooms. Neither could a tailor properly measure Gulliver for a suit; using abstract formulas rather than simple measurements of length, in six days the tailor returned with clothes that were completely misshapen. They even had trouble attending to people right in front of them, so distracted were they by their abstract thought. That's why all the Laputan nobility were accompanied by "flappers," servants who carried a kind of rattle at the end of a long stick to "flap" the Laputans on the ears whenever someone wanted to talk to them.[32] Caught up in their internal world of what they calculated to be true, the truth of real people and concrete things was easily lost.

Could that be us one day? Or is it already partially true? The neutral view, as helpful as it can be, when it loses contact with embodied life, is no longer connected to real people in particular circumstances. For too long we have misunderstood this powerful reinterpretation of reality brought about by the statistical gaze. Not the fault of numbers that reveal reality, we are increasingly crunching numbers to change reality, crushing our view of self and of one another at the same time.

If we are to continue to learn from the science of probability and statistics, we must set aside the idiosyncrasies of the particular for the sake of the universal. But in putting the particular aside, we must honestly face the great and grave possibility that our temporary forgetfulness becomes a permanent loss of memory. For the particular is with us only in fragile form, easily vanishing in the mist of abstract numbering and objectified life. To firmly grasp the beauty of the particular knitted together with all its parts—aside from our own individually assigned "flapper"—we need a way of seeing that refuses to make the person in front of us an abstract and fixed image of our own making. To remain open to the rarity and marvel of the person before us, we need a hope made possible by faith.

6

The Gaze of the Gospel

The Incarnation invites me to seek the face of God in the
face of everybody whom I encounter.

Ivan Illich

There is a Chinese proverb that says "two-thirds of what we see is
behind our eyes." Aside from showing that attempts to calculate the
incalculable is not confined to Western culture, more importantly it
reminds us that a significant proportion of our perception is formed
before we ever look. Today's health care encounter is filled with pre-
conceived notions heavily influenced by the disembodied gaze. Consider how what you see is influenced by what you already take for
granted in the following scenarios.

In one room is a patient with recurrent liver disease who drinks
too much. Since this happens over and over, you already know that
your efforts to help him will fall on deaf ears. In another is someone
who always has a list complaints, none ever specific enough to lead to
a diagnosis— you've learned that ordering tests is just a waste of time
and money because the results are always normal. The third patient
has diabetes, hypertension, and family history of colon cancer. There
are over ten boxes to check if you are to complete the recommended

management of her diseases and risks—you can only hope she has no concerns or questions, because you have time only to do what you already know she needs. You find out the last patient is angry because your treatment from the previous visit gave him no help for his pain. You brace yourself for an unpleasant visit—you already know that no matter what you do, this patient will be dissatisfied with your care.

Prepped with preexisting information and past behavior, most current-day practitioners quickly cram patients into categories of diagnosis, statistical risk, or fixed behavior. At one level, it makes the work manageable by allowing the great number of people needing help to more quickly fit into known plans of care. But the abstraction of people, either fractured into their parts via the clinical gaze or melded into a population via the statistical gaze, is also one of the greatest dangers in health care, if not in our culture. The person that lies in a hospital bed or waits in the exam room is silently hoping, "Please, see me!"; the health care team, as much as they desire to care for you as a particular embodied person, cannot help but see you as a fixed package of problems and potential diseases, a dissected body created by the medical gaze.

Rescuing the body is "one of the deepest unresolved issues of our modern Western culture."[1] To gain from the knowledge of clinical understanding or statistical evaluation but not lose sight of the particular embodied patient is a difficult task indeed. Surrounded by reductive forces, we need another way of seeing. It must be a good and strong gaze if it is to hold the pattern of the whole together, seeing each one as unique creation. It would require training of the eye and ongoing practice, akin to the skilled appraiser of art who has learned to look at a work and know if it is an original. And it would be a fragile thing, fleeting and easily stolen away by the power of other views that tell lies about the authenticity or value of the artwork. Up against all these challenges, the good news is that it is actually possible.

The Gaze of the Gospel

The word *gospel* means "glad tidings" or "good news."[2] Attached to orthodox Christian understanding, it is the astounding news that God chose to become like us and accept life in a human body, realized in the birth of Jesus Christ to a young girl named Mary. While both the promise of his coming and the fulfillment of it are found throughout the whole Bible, perhaps the most succinct summary is found in a little verse in the small book of Colossians: "In Christ all the fullness of the Deity lives in bodily form" (Col. 2:9).

So much said in so few words: God, the Creator of all things, including the human race, became one of us. How can that be? It is like the potter becoming like one of the clay artifacts she has made. It is the miracle above all others, or as C. S. Lewis called it, the "one grand miracle . . . that what is beyond all space and time, what is uncreated, eternal, came into nature, descended into His own universe."[3] If it is hard to understand, be assured you are in large company: of the things Christians believe, the incarnation, God in-carnate, embodied in human flesh, is the most distinct, decisive, and challenging of all. Yet whatever else it is, from the moment it happened, it was meant to be good news, heard clearly in the angel's announcement to shepherds out in a field on that quiet night: "Do not be afraid. I bring you good news that willl cause great joy for all the people. Today in the town of David a Savior has been born to you; he is the Messiah, the Lord" (Luke 2:10–11).

To fully explain why Jesus Christ coming in human form is good news extends far beyond the boundaries of this book or the capabilities of this author. But amidst the richness of this reality, we will explore two ideas that are germane to our purpose. First, good news or not, the incarnation is surely disorienting news for everyone who hears it, so strange that it is easily drowned out in the more natural noise of everyday life. Second, because God came in a human body, a new perception of the body is offered; seeing ourselves and others in the light of the incarnation may even require a change in the way we pursue health and practice health care.

The Surprise and Fragility of the Incarnation

After about four hundred years of silence between the Old and New Testaments, the announcement that God would appear to his people again, in the form of a little baby born to an inconsequential teenager who wasn't even married yet, in a wooden manger in a small village

called Bethlehem, was a shocking thought. No one could have anticipated such an entrance—and a lot of angels were dispatched so that
it might be heard. Initial reactions were far and wide, from perplexity, acceptance, and gratitude to anger, disbelief, fear, and opposition.
Coming this gently, this softly, this weakly, it was unsettling to anyone's conception of God.

Three individuals in the biblical narrative show how unexpected it
was. Zechariah was a priest, married to Elizabeth, both of them old
and beyond hope of having a child. An angel visited him one day in
the temple. When told they would have a son who would prepare the
way for the coming of God, it was too much for him to accept. Struck
dumb for his disbelief, he was unable to speak for many months. But
his days of silence were not in vain. On the day the angel's words
came true, Zechariah's speech returned; recognizing that his son, John,
would indeed be a prophet of God (he became John the Baptist), he
lifted his voice and proclaimed the good news that the Lord was coming to rescue his people.[4]

Mary was confused and afraid when the angel Gabriel first greeted
her with the news that God had a special plan for her. Then he told her
that she would bear a son, even as a virgin, and that she was to give
him the name Jesus. "He will be great and will be called the Son of the
Most High. The Lord God will give him the throne of his father David,
and he will reign over Jacob's descendants forever; his kingdom will
never end" (Luke 1:31–33). She, unlike Zechariah initially, received
this extraordinary announcement with humility and trust.

Finally there was Herod, the king of Judea. It was not a divine visitation but wise men from the east, who told him a king would be born
within his domain. Never considering this could be heaven coming to
earth, he saw it only as a political threat to his own rule. His plan was
to kill the child, ultimately leading to the death of many little boys in
Bethlehem in his attempt to eradicate this delicate entrance of God
into the world.[5] From this odd and vulnerable beginning, the surprise
and fragility of the incarnation has continued ever since.

After the death of Christ, the incarnation came under immediate
attack in the Greco-Roman world of the first and second centuries.
Heavily influenced by a neoplatonic dualism that saw spirit and matter

as separate, the thought of the divine nature being embodied in sordid and lowly human flesh was nonsense. To denounce this preposterous idea, Gnosticism, as already described, quickly rose up and grew in a variety of sects. The first Christians realized how easily belief in the incarnation could be snuffed out by the prevailing forces. Cherishing its importance, they entered a fight for its survival, counted by many to be the hardest and most decisive battle in church history.[6]

Of the many early church leaders who considered the mystery of the incarnation central to Christianity, none stood with more focus and determination than Irenaeus, bishop of Lyons, born in Asia Minor around AD 125. Knowing the ease with which every generation to follow would try to marginalize the incarnation, he confronted the false teaching of Gnosticism with the pure claim that Jesus was God made man.

> But, according to these men, neither was the Word made flesh, nor Christ, nor the Saviour. . . . For they will have it, that the Word and Christ never came into this world; that the Saviour, too, never became incarnate, nor suffered. . . . For if anyone carefully examines the systems of them all, he will find that the Word of God is brought in by all of them as not having become incarnate. . . . Therefore the Lord's disciple, pointing them all out as false witnesses, says, "And the Word was made flesh, and dwelt among us" (John 1:14).[7]

As many have done since, Irenaeus returned over and over to the first chapter of John, written by "the Lord's disciple" who was one of Jesus's closest friends, to defend the truth of the incarnation. Refusing to accept any Gnostic attempts to denigrate the body,[8] in one of his most famous phrases he called the body "doubly good." Made good in creation, as we noted when discussing Genesis 1, corruption followed our fall in the garden; but in the incarnation the goodness of the body is restored once again and for all time.

In the fleeting vision of the incarnation, always under threat by the reductive forces of every age, the restoration of the body as a good gift offers us a new way of seeing. By the power of this perception we have the potential to change for good the way we pursue health and practice health care. It is to the implications of the incarnation for health (focusing on how we see ourselves) and for health care (focusing on how we see others) that we now turn.

A Body You Have Prepared for Me

When God chose to come to the world embodied in Jesus Christ, he accepted life with all of its limitations, from his dependence on his mother Mary as an infant, to the ups and downs of adolescence, the need for food and sleep, the susceptibility to sickness, the inevitability of suffering, and the experience of death. Apart from these more obvious realities of life in a body, at the heart of the biblical vision of the incarnation is that the time, place, family, and particular body that Jesus inhabited were not a random accident but designed for the sake of his specific destiny. Jesus knew that everything about his earthly life, including the body he inhabited, was to fulfill God's intended purpose. In the following passage we gain a glimpse of Jesus's self-understanding of his mission:

> Sacrifice and offering you did not desire, but a body you prepared for me. . . . Then I said, "Here I am—it is written about me in the scroll—I have come to do your will, my God." (Heb. 10:5, 7)

In that statement, destiny and the body are melded together in an inseparable unity in Jesus Christ, linking the concrete form of his life with the work he was sent to do. Accepting that this applies to the great and glorious mission of the Son of God, who is the Savior of the world, is a big thought; it becomes even bigger and much more personal when we extend it to every one of us as fellow embodied creatures. Let's look at three consequences of seeing the body as gift and intimately connected to our destiny.

First, despite all our efforts to escape the body and seek salvation apart from it, the enduring fact is that God's plan of redemption for us will not be apart from the body but in, through, and for the body. Second, the particular form of our body, including the measure of health we have and the place and time in which we live, is not accidental but filled with potential purpose. Finally, the frailty and finitude of our body represents not extraneous limitation but an intentional part of the gift that is our body. To illustrate some of what this means, let's look at a fictional story, a living example, and a common scenario.

In Robertson Davies's novel *The Rebel Angels*, Ozy Froats, a renowned but unpretentious scientist, is having a discussion about body types with Simon Darcourt, a priest. Simon has been hoping that by diet and exercise he would be able to moderate his tendency toward a round, chunky body. When he asks his scientist friend if he thinks it is possible, Ozy speaks more soberly:

> To some extent. Not without more trouble than it would probably be worth. That's what's wrong with all these diets and body-building courses and so forth. . . . The body is the inescapable factor, you see. You can keep in good shape for what you are, but radical change is impossible. Health isn't making everybody into a Greek ideal; it's living out the destiny of your body. . . . But it isn't simple, being yourself. . . . They get some mental picture of themselves and then they devil the poor old body, trying to make it like the picture. When it won't obey—can't obey, of course—they are mad at it and live in it as if it were an unsatisfactory house they were hoping to move out of. A lot of illness comes from that.[9]

If our bodies are an inescapable fact, then trying to change them beyond what they are meant to be is likely to make us sick rather than healthy. This in no way dismisses or discredits a thoughtful care of the body that includes healthy diet, good exercise, and proper rest. But if the form of our body is not incidental but essential, the sooner we embrace our body, the sooner we embrace our destiny—as someone like Randy does every day.

Randy, a man in his fifties, was born with cerebral palsy and has been confined to a wheelchair all his life. A patient at the health center for over twenty years, on one of his recent visits he was thanking us profusely for our help in getting him a new chair. He was overjoyed and infectiously shared with childlike wonder how the new turn signals and backup lights improved his confidence as he traversed the sidewalks and streets of the city. Though Randy often has needs, he is never needy. Intelligent and thoughtful, yet able to move only his upper body with any control, he has never seen his limitations as disabling. He is engaged in life, a leader in his church, and a manager in the apartment building where he lives in community with others having similar challenges. Above all, Randy doesn't see his life as limited by function, but controlled by purpose; he is always excited about the next new thing that he can do to aid his neighbor or serve his God. Without any plan to do so, he inspires almost everyone he meets.

Lastly, we face the increasingly pertinent question, "What do we do with all the choices we have to change our body?" Cosmetically, we can alter ourselves to be more culturally beautiful or socially acceptable. Physically, we can gain strength by increasing our muscle mass with steroids, change the oxygen-carrying capacity of our blood for greater endurance with erythropoietin, or juice ourselves with stimulants for more energy—all so that we can perform at higher levels and achieve greater accomplishments. More radically, we can even change our gender with hormones and sex-reassignment surgery.

Perhaps you easily dismiss as extreme most of these measures to change your looks or how you perform; but what if altering the body could reduce the risk of disease? Many organs harbor a future risk of cancer, and some have chosen to remove those organs—a breast or a colon, for example—to remove that risk. Depending on the risk, the organ, and the age, this may be wise in limited cases. But what about my young friend who has Lynch syndrome, an inherited genetic variant that increases the risk of several cancers over her lifetime? Highest is an 80 percent risk of colon cancer, but she also has a significantly increased risk of stomach cancer, liver cancer, endometrial cancer, and ovarian cancer. How many body parts should she remove? Some have advised her to have her colon, uterus, and ovaries removed before it's too late, though she is only in her twenties, unmarried, and with no children.[10]

If our bodies are little more than two-legged bundles of potential disease, then that is exactly what she should do. But if a life embodied is always a risk, and the destiny of our lives is connected to the body we have been given, embracing our purpose becomes more important than escaping risk. Such perceptions bring new possibilities for life in the body and the purpose of health care. If meaning and purpose are deeply tied to the very form and fit of our body, then our task and the task of medicine must advance beyond the blunt power to free ourselves from the limitations of our body to learning to live in and through the bodies we have been given.

I See an Image

The incarnation astounds for many reasons, and its implications for how we see our body and pursue health are great. But there is another meaning of the incarnation that is even more remarkable: to dare to think that through the person in front of us we may encounter God. Rooted in our creation in God's image, as previously discussed, in the gaze of the gospel we are offered the invitation to see the face of God in our neighbor, particularly our neighbor in need. This latter perspective is brought out in sharpest contrast by a conversation that Jesus had with his friends shortly before his death. Describing a judgment scene at the end of time (Matt. 25:31–46), the critical question for each one is whether they fed Jesus when he was hungry, gave him drink when he was thirsty, clothed him when he was naked, visited him when he was sick or in prison, or invited him in when he was a stranger. All are incredulous because none can understand when they ever saw Jesus in these circumstances. Then in one of the most dramatic statements in the Bible, Jesus says, "Truly I tell you, whatever you did [or did not do] for one of the least of these brothers and sisters of mine, you did [or did not do] for me" (Matt. 25:40, 45).

From thinking that showing hospitality to strangers is akin to entertaining angels (Heb. 13:2), to a radical change in the way the early church saw and responded to the sick,[11] to believing that only through the eyes of the suffering will we see a true view of the world,[12] the influence of that idea on the history of Christianity is immeasurable. To recover some of the power of this gaze for our own time, let's consider several ways this view may influence the practice of health care today.

A bias toward love. If the person before us is both made in God's image and uniquely loved by God, then whatever the good, the bad, the beautiful, or the ugly that we first see when we look, we are biased toward love. Many fellow human beings can be quite lovely, but many others are not; and everyone is unlovely at one time or another. But if our vision is rooted in the gaze of the gospel, then our love has life beyond any feeling, circumstance, or assessment of value, except in knowing that the person is valued by God. As Dietrich Bonhoeffer wrote:

> Only because God became human is it possible to know and not despise real human beings. . . . This is not because of the real human being's inherent value, but because God has loved and taken on the real human being. The reason for God's love for human beings does not reside in them, but only in God. Our living as real human beings, and loving the real people next to us is, again, grounded only in God's becoming human, in the unfathomable love of God for us human beings.[13]

An appreciation of the particular. This love for the person brought about by the gaze of the gospel cannot help but bring about a greater interest in, appreciation for, and protection of the particularities of their life. The distinct quality of love is that it "is never abstract. It does not adhere to the universe or the planet or the nation or the institution or the profession, but to the singular sparrows of the street, the lilies of the field, 'the least of these my brethren.'"[14] In love, the particular person cannot be treated as any person. And when we need to know if someone is well, or if sick, what will help him to get better, loving particular people in particular circumstances offers a means of assessment far more precise than the accuracy of measured outcomes or statistical indicators.

An openness to surprise. In contrast to approaching people with knowledge gained through diagnosis, sociological categorization, or imputed needs, the gaze of the gospel moves us beyond fixed relationships into the domain of contingency. Rather than fearing what we cannot control or predict, we wonder if God may show up in the next person we meet. It may be the noncompliant diabetic patient who for the first time has decided to exercise more and take her medications correctly, or the alcoholic patient who has stopped drinking and wants to start over, or the chronically sad patient who for once has some hope. In each case, like the dry branch that you thought dead and would now cut off, new life suddenly springs up in the strangest places. Even small things may have great value, as the following example of a tired doctor seeing a last patient shows.

It was the end of a long day, and the doctor had agreed to see one more patient because she was a relative of a staff member. When the doctor heard that the patient was the staff member's grandmother, a new patient, and ninety-two years old, he quickly regretted his decision; a new, elderly patient always has a long list of problems, and it was already after hours. He entered the room expecting the worst and felt verified when he saw the patient, her daughter, and her granddaughter, assuming each one had her own list of concerns. Instead, they told him that there were no problems; actually, this matriarch of the family didn't even know why she needed to see a doctor at all, but because they cherished her so much she agreed to come.

Feeling relieved, he quickly confirmed that she was doing well, recommended a few basic blood tests, and got up to leave. But not yet—suddenly the patient, who had been quiet and passive while the family did most of the talking, now spoke up and asked for one more thing. At first he didn't grasp what she was saying; was it because of his limited Spanish, or because he couldn't believe what he thought she said? So he turned to the family, who confirmed it: she wanted to pray for him. With surprisingly quick and firm actions, she moved close, placed her hands on his head, and proceeded to pronounce a rural Mexican blessing over him, asking God to protect him, to use him to be a healer in people's lives, and to give him love for his patients and strength to endure for many more years. Far beyond what the doctor expected, the good of this visit only became clear at the last minute and in a completely unanticipated direction, which brings us to our final point.

The movement of the Spirit in two directions. The gaze of the gospel, by biasing us toward love of the particular and opening us to surprise, turns the person in front of us from a fixed image of our own making to an image of God that makes every encounter potentially sacred. We pause in such a moment and, in our recognition of the dignity and respect that each deserves, invite unforeseen possibilities for hope and healing. And what greater surprise could there be, while seeking the goodness of God in your life, that the person who is changed most is me.

The way God comes to us in the incarnation was, is, and always will be a surprise, a pure gift beyond expectation or understanding. Only by faith can we look for things beyond comprehension, and even then, in the face of harsher realities, it is often but a fragile impression or a fleeting glimmer, as T. S. Eliot reminds us:

> These are only hints and guesses,
> Hints followed by guesses; and the rest
> Is prayer, observance, discipline, thought and action.
> The hint half-guessed, the gift half understood, is
> Incarnation.[15]

For some, it is foolishness even to try. But with observation, discipline, thought, action, and prayer, we will experience moments that will sustain us in an embodied practice of health care, helping us to keep the tapestry together no matter how strong the forces that are pulling the threads apart. It is hard work, really an impossible task—until we see Randy and are reminded how little it has to do with us. People like Randy reverse the flow, with the glow of the gospel in him teaching everyone he meets that how we see ourselves, and how we see each other, has little to do with the way the parts of our body function or whether they obey the statistical rules, and everything to do with how God sees us. And that is a gaze worth nurturing.

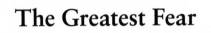

The Greatest Fear

7

In the Shadow of Death

[God] has also set eternity in the human heart.

Ecclesiastes 3:11

As no one has power over the wind to contain it,
so no one has power over the time of their death.

Ecclesiastes 8:8

There was a certain man who enjoyed good health. In fact, his health was very good. As he grew older he decided to improve his health with regular exercise, eventually working out two hours a day. Friends told him he was in excellent shape, much more than most his age, so he decided to enter some competitive races. With each event he performed at higher levels. He even ran a twenty-six-mile marathon and finished in the top 10 percent for his age. He thought to himself, "I am in very good shape and enjoy the best of health. I wish to protect it in every way possible and want to be strong all my years. I will get the colonoscopy and vaccinations my doctor recommended. But I will also get a total body scan. Since the advertisment promises it will check everything, then I can be sure I will stay healthy." He got all the tests, and they all came back normal, so he said to himself, "I have many years of good things laid out for me. Be happy and content. Tomorrow I will sign up for another marathon, work out three hours a day, and do even better than last year." But that night he died.[1]

And therein lies the rub: we desire to live a long and healthy life but cannot avoid the fact that our death is an ultimate necessity and continual possibility. As the writer of Ecclesiastes says, we desire eternity but cannot even control the day of our death. Posing it as a dilemma, as all wise teachers do, it leaves us longing for an answer. But the crux of our problem is not our mortality; all living creatures share that fate. Our predicament is that we are "thinking reeds," as seventeenth-century religious philosopher and mathematician Blaise Pascal describes us, and for that reason uniquely aware of how fragile life is:

> Man is only a reed, the feeblest thing in nature, but, he is a thinking reed. It is not necessary for the entire universe to take up arms in order to crush him. A vapour, a drop of water, is sufficient to kill him. But if the universe crushed him, man would still be nobler than the thing which destroys him, because he knows he is dying, and the universe which has him at its mercy is unaware of it.[2]

Does it make us nobler to know that we are dying, as Pascal assumed? Or are we overwhelmed by our insecurities in the shadow of death, resigned either to frightful denial, friendly embrace, or fight to the bitter end? But if we choose not to run from it, passively accept it, or rage against it, what else is there?

What is to be explored in this chapter is how we deal with the persistent shadow of death in a society that has eroded its domain more than any preceding age or culture—after all, Pascal's drop of water is much less dangerous in an age of public hygiene. But if recent success is giving us fresh hope that we are about to escape its shadow, we should remember how long people have been trying to run from death. The desire to overcome death is a very old dream, a dream as old as humanity itself.

Timeless Questions

Let us go back to the oldest of stories, to one of the world's first great epics, the Epic of Gilgamesh, composed in Babylonia more than three thousand years ago. Gilgamesh is thought to have been a historical king who reigned in the Sumerian city of Uruk in Mesopotamia (now Iraq) in about 2750 BC. In the way the story is told, the king is part god and part man. "Surpassing all kings," his mighty feats in battle and great success building up the city have made him famous; but it also made him a tyrant who is uncaring and abusive of his people.[3]

So the people cry out to heaven for help, and the gods hear their plea. They create a new hero, Enkidu, whose strength and courage will balance Gilgamesh and bring peace to Uruk. On first meeting they fight for supremacy, and the king overcomes Enkidu. But a mutual respect is formed that forges a friendship unlike any the king has ever known.

In search of greater fame, the king convinces Enkidu to go out with him on his adventures, believing that together they will be invincible. They meet creatures of mythic proportions, winning every battle. But their conquests, ill-conceived and arrogant, have offended the gods. Enkidu becomes ill, and over twelve long days, despite the prayers of his friend, he weakens and dies.

> When he heard the death rattle, Gilgamesh moaned
> like a dove. His face grew dark. "Beloved,
> wait, don't leave me. Dearest of men,
> don't die, don't let them take you from me."
> All through the long night, Gilgamesh wept
> For his dear friend.[4]

At this point the story takes a dramatic turn. His grief at the loss of his friend suddenly turns to a preoccupation with his own death:

> Must I die too? Must I be as lifeless
> as Enkidu? How can I bear this sorrow
> that gnaws at my belly, this fear of death
> that restlessly drives me onward?[5]

Driven by anguish and fear, Gilgamesh sets out on a desperate search for immortality. Along the way he meets many obstacles and dangers, but none are a match for the power of his obsession. At one point he meets a friendly figure; seeing the strain he is under, she gently counsels him to abandon his futile quest in favor of a finite life:

> Gilgamesh, where are you roaming?
> You will never find the eternal life
> that you seek. When the gods created mankind,
> they also created death, and they held back
> eternal life for themselves alone.
> Humans are born, they live, they die,
> this is the order that the gods have decreed.[6]

But Gilgamesh receives no comfort from the inevitability of death:

> Enkidu, my brother, whom I loved so dearly,
> who accompanied me through every danger—
> the fate of mankind has overwhelmed him.
> For six days I would not let him be buried,
> thinking, "If my grief is violent enough,
> perhaps he will come back to life." . . .
> Then I was frightened, I was terrified by death,
> and I set out to roam the wilderness.
> I cannot bear what happened to my friend—
> I cannot bear what happened to Enkidu—
> so I roam the wilderness in grief.
> How can my mind find rest?
> My beloved friend has turned into clay—
> my beloved Enkidu has turned into clay.
> And won't I too lie down in the dirt
> like him, and never arise again?[7]

The questions and quests of thousands of years have changed little over the centuries. The anguish in loss, fear of death, and desire for immortality run like deep and disturbing waters throughout human history. Harkening back to our discussion of Genesis, from the moment we chose the Tree of Knowledge and left the garden, we have been trying to get back to the Tree of Life. We cannot escape our desire for immortality, placed deep within us in our creation. But neither can we forget the self-conscious knowledge of mortality we received the moment we were separated from life in the garden. Ernest Becker, in his Pulitzer Prize–winning book, *The Denial of Death*, describes our emergence from the garden in this way:

> Man emerged . . . and came to reflect on his condition. He was given a consciousness of his individuality and his part-divinity in creation, the beauty and uniqueness of his face and his name. At the same time he was given the consciousness of the terror of the world and his own death and decay. This paradox is the really constant thing about man in all periods of history and society; it is thus the true "essence" of man.[8]

Further on he describes this paradoxical "essence of man" more fully:

> What does it mean to be a self-conscious animal? The idea is ludicrous, if it is not monstrous. It means to know that one is food for worms. This is the terror: to have emerged from nothing, to have a name, consciousness of self, deep inner feelings, an excruciating inner yearning for life and self-expression—and with all this yet to die.[9]

Afflicted by the self-conscious dread that we are food for worms, our deepest need is to be free of the anxiety of death. Consequently our whole life and all that we do, Becker says, is to drive death from our conscious lives. Stuck in our choice for independence and control, from time immemorial we have been making our quests to escape death on our own terms and by our own devices. The pursuit of the Holy Grail is nothing new; the only thing that changes is the paths we pursue and the options we have.

Immortalism Today

Evidence of our desire to "live long and prosper" appears in many forms in our day and age. The most sensational remind us of the heroic quests of the past, really more conquest than quest; recent covers of *Time* magazine forecast immortality around the corner,[10] billions of dollars are being poured into regenerative medicine in the hope of significantly expanding the human life span, and cryonics are freezing bodies to await future rejuvenation by our more medically sophisticated descendants.[11] If hopes to end death through nanotechnology, gene therapy, and artificial intelligence seem fantastic, futuristic, and far away, closer to home we can find signs of immortalism in the form and function of everyday health care. Some examples include the following.

The dominance of battle imagery in our struggle with disease. Our language betrays our intentions. We are currently waging a "war" on cancer, "conquering" disease, "overcoming" aging, and using our "weapons" of technology to "take back territory" from death. The battle lines are drawn, and we expect to "win" the fight and claim the "victory."

A tendency toward optimistic prognostications. Most doctors and nurses find it difficult to tell patients the truth about their prognosis, often overestimating how much time the patient has left. In one commonly cited study of terminally ill patients that assessed the ability of 365 doctors to determine prognosis, most predictions were overly optimistic; overall patients were told they would live five times longer than they actually did. The doctors who knew their patients better were more likely to overestimate the survival of their patients than those less involved in the patients' lives.[12] Though this evidence may be the result of genuine sensitivity, it also reveals a personal hesitancy to face the truth about mortality with those we know best.[13]

Skewed Medicare spending. Nearly 30 percent of Medicare expenditures occur in the last six months of life,[14] with more than half of that amount spent in the last month.[15] Unfortunately, much of this spending occurs for care in hospitals and intensive care units, meaning that too many of a person's last days are spent hooked to monitors and tubes, receiving "high tech" care that at best delays death for a short time rather than extending life for a meaningful period.

Patient expectations. When asked about end-of-life decisions, a growing number of people in the United States say that medical professionals should always do everything possible to keep patients alive.[16] Simple and self-evident in most other contexts, at the end of life it is a burdensome expectation in light of how much can be done already and how much more will be possible in the future. Even a working religious faith does not automatically increase mindfulness of mortality and decrease dependence on lifesaving treatment when death is imminent; counter to expectations, in some cases this group of people was more likely to request aggressive treatments at the end of life.[17] For many with religious commitments, options for sustaining life are equated with a moral requirement to use them. Making the fight against death a test of personal devotion, technology becomes an unadulterated and dependable ally in the struggle.[18]

All these signs, and there are many more, point to three unique components of our current struggle with mortality. First, we are resting our dreams for immortality more and more upon the promises of biotechnology. That this is true should not surprise us, as it has been a desire of the scientific enterprise since its origins, as bioethicist Leon Kass explains it:

> For truth to tell, victory over mortality is the unstated but implicit goal of modern medical science, indeed of the entire modern scientific project, to which mankind was summoned almost four hundred years ago by Francis Bacon and René Descartes. They quite consciously trumpeted the conquest of nature for the relief of man's estate, and they founded a science whose explicit purpose was to reverse the curse laid on Adam and Eve, and especially to restore the tree of life, by means of the tree of (scientific) knowledge. With medicine's increasing successes, realized mainly in the last half-century, every death is increasingly regarded as premature, a failure of today's medicine that future research will prevent.[19]

Failing to remember that our days are numbered with "limits [we] cannot exceed" (Job 14:5), death in this new context becomes a correctable biological deficiency, with biotechnology giving us the tools to fix it.[20]

Second, despite our efforts to show death the door, it has come back in through the window, requiring us to develop two modern ways to manage the scandal of its persistence: either we silence it as taboo, banishing it from daily life, or we accept it as a technical fact, reducing it to the state of an ordinary thing.[21] In the former case we make it shameful, treating death "with much the same prudery as the sexual impulses were a century ago."[22] As something indecent and dirty, it offends our sense of modesty. So we hide it behind the sterile sheets of a hospital bed or use the skills of the mortician to remove its distasteful decay, maintaining the appearance of life for the sake of the living who long ago ceased to tolerate its sights, sounds, or smells.[23] In the latter case, we reduce it to something as insignificant as it is necessary. Quite the opposite of the taboo, we speak of death openly, but as if of little importance; with little emotion, we respect the natural dignity of the dying but in detached and efficient tones. In neither case is the power and ugliness of death confronted or the depth of loss acknowledged or displays of mourning supported. In both cases it is discreet, clean, and quiet, leaving on tiptoe, making no sound, undisturbing to larger society so that the rest of us can get on with our duty "to look well, to seem fine, and to exclude from the fabric of his or her normal life any evidence of decay and death and helplessness."[24]

Third, the desire for personal control over one's life and death, present for many decades prior, has of late become an almost obsessive preoccupation. As bioethicist Daniel Callahan suggests, nothing seems to be more feared than loss of self-determination:

> As death has been drained of social meaning, the right to control the conditions of dying has been all the more strongly asserted. The demand for control, the unwillingness to accept death as it might present itself untouched, is not only strong, it has become a passion for many. The only evil greater than one's personal death is increasingly taken to be the loss of control of that death.[25]

Through this lens of control, we can better understand behaviors at the end of life that might seem, at first blush, inconsistent. On one end, there is an anxious affirmation of earthly life—in the hours and days that precede our death, despite all evidence that our numbered days are over, we wedge ourselves into unlikely spaces and hang on, hoping for a medical miracle or a sudden turn of events. On the other end, there seems an indifferent contempt of this life—when we tire of it, we want the right to end it, and, taking back control from a medical system that would force life-prolonging technology on us, we demand the power to choose when and how we will die.[26] The power to discontinue, like the power to prolong, is cut from the same cloth: the desire to control the hour of our death.

Clearly, we are ambivalent about our companionship with modern medical technology in our struggle to live with our mortality. Yet with no larger meaning or wider context for death and dying, whatever means increases our control, either delaying it until later or choosing it now, gives a sense of victory. But the more we fear death and seek to run from it or confront death with the liberating force of our right to choose it, the more buried and hidden is the meaning of death in our lives. How did we come to have such a sterile view of death?

The Disenchantment of the Universe

Finding meaning in death, a challenge for any age, has become particularly difficult in a world no longer full of "charged things," or what Charles Taylor calls "the disenchantment of the universe."[27] A multilayered process taking place over much time and passing through several stages, we will confine ourselves to the simple comparison between then and now.

Five hundred years ago the world was seen as an enchanted cosmos, full of spirits, demons, and moral forces. It was a world of meaning outside human control, full of things charged with causal power. This context allowed a greater acceptance of death as part of life and a heightened awareness of when death was approaching.[28] The saints and heroic figures of the period were revered for their ability to sense the time was near, having a "premonition of death and the way in which it is deeply rooted in daily life."[29] From the way that knights such as King Ban die in Arthurian legends—"He looked up at heaven and said as well as he could. . . . 'O Lord God . . . help me, for I see and I know that my end has come'"[30]—to pious monks who knew that death was near—"He saw death standing beside him and knew that he was about to die"[31]—the ability to sense death's arrival and prepare accordingly were the actions of the wise and honorable. On the contrary, to avoid death's warning and attempt to cheat death exposed one to ridicule, with the literature of that day mocking a perverse and unrealistic attachment to this life. As one biographer summed up his admiration for a peasant family's ability to discern the time: "We see how (they) in those bygone days passed from this world to the next simply and straightforwardly observing the signs, and above all, observing themselves. They were in no hurry to die, but when they saw the time approaching, then not too soon and not too late, but just when they were supposed to, they died like Christians."[32] Then, as now, in the undiscovered country that is the end of our lives, there was a time to fight and a time to surrender; the important thing was to be sensitive to the signs.

The ability to "simply and straightforwardly observe the signs" is the stuff of bygone days, according to Taylor, because we live in an age closed to outside power. Enclosed within the "immanent frame," time has no meaning beyond measured units that move in a single dimension of before, now, and after. Long gone are sacred dimensions that gathered, assembled, and reordered ordinary time, allowing the expression of higher reality in the things that surround us.[33] Time simply advances in uniform chronology—we may use it as a simple commodity or protect it as a precious resource, but in neither case is it open to heightened moments of special revelation. Aided by the Enlightenment view of nature's strict order, signs and wonder disappear in a mechanized world, leaving a disenchanted universe of objective reality that can be studied, understood, and exploited. The mystery of death, as all mystery, is voided—in a flattened space and time organized into discrete and analyzable problems, there is no place for it.

While much has been gained, much has been lost in the disenchantment that dissolved the cosmos of meaningful causal forces. No longer able to see God as an active agent in the world—at best an architect of an ordered universe, at worst a vestige of a childish view of the world—we can no longer sense the signs of approaching death, as our ancestors did,[34] nor do we believe that life in its arc from birth to death contains God's actions of preservation and provision. Lacking confidence in the goodness of present life bounded by a beginning and an end, we are more aware than ever that underneath our enlightened view of order and control remains the random chaos of a hostile universe of accidents and genetic mutations. No matter how unlikely the events we fear, we live in the shadow of death because no one is acting for our good in the impersonal universe that we inhabit. Nor can we hear when our time is at end, because the universe is quiet—what Camus named *le silence déraisonnable du monde* (the unreasonable silence of the world).[35] The only sound is the ticking clock of a mechanically ordered universe. And just as a clock endlessly goes round and round, we are tempted to believe we can continually prolong our days if only we have the right tools for fixing our personal timepiece.

Does Anybody Know What Time It Is?

Has the universe gone silent? Or are the sounds just more subtle? And if there are still discerning ears to hear, it may be only in unexpected places that we will find them.

Margaret had been a recent admission to Cook County Hospital for a cough and weight loss. As a resident on the hospital service at the largest public hospital in Chicago, I was responsible for the care of indigent patients sent up from the emergency room. I discussed the case with the team, ordered the usual tests, and by the third day knew that she had inoperable lung cancer. After consulting with oncology, I went to explain her diagnosis and treatment.

Though aware of the grave prognosis, I was buoyed by the options for treatment and believed that I could instill hope into an otherwise despairing situation by carefully explaining her choices. When I arrived at her room, she seemed oblivious to what was coming—she happily showed off the braids in her hair that her granddaughter had done that morning and asked how I was doing, which was her usual custom. I sat down and told her I had bad news. I plunged forward with the sad facts, quickly interjected the hopeful range of treatments available, and braced myself for her response.

But I was not ready for what she said. She told me she had assumed something like this was what she had. Then she thanked me for the careful evaluation of her problems, asked if she could continue the medicines that were helping her pain, and said she was ready to go home. I was shocked at what I was sure was a bad decision. I even felt anger that she would reject the potent treatment we could give her. I told her bluntly she would die soon if she went home and asked her to reconsider all that we could do for her. I even asked her to think about her family and how much they would miss her. And after listening carefully to each and every thing I said, in the briefest of words but firm and full of meaning, she said, "It is time for me to go home." She left the hospital and died in peace amidst the love of family three months later.

How did this uneducated woman, who had lived most of her life picking cotton in rural Mississippi and was now sitting in a hospital bed in Chicago with metastatic lung cancer, know what time it was? I thought about her advanced cancer. I looked at my own hope in treatment that could only extend her life a short time and perhaps with many complications. And I saw that she had a unique understanding of life forged through years of struggle and poverty that made her dependent on God. She knew something I didn't know, aware of time and sensitive to signs that I was not trained to see.

It has always been difficult to discern the time. But our willingness to listen will only begin with faith that someone is speaking. I believe Margaret would say it is worth the effort, because it is a voice that speaks peace to an anxious age, when we are healthy and fear an unknown future, or when we are dying and wonder what is next. I am convinced that the way we live and listen now will inform the way we die later. If we train our ears, perhaps when the day comes we will be prepared to hear the sounds, observe the signs, and know the time. And if there is no time and we have no warning, even still we will be ready.

But before we can "interpret the signs of the times" today, we must first wrestle with a bewildering and significant event in the past: the Son of God in a grave for three days.[36]

8

Death Defanged and Defeated

I am not in danger: only near to death.

Thomas, in *Murder in the Cathedral*[1]

Archbishop Thomas Becket and the king of England are at odds with each other. The king is angry that this godly man is threatening his earthly power. Seeking to please the king and gain glory for themselves, four knights go to Canterbury to kill the archbishop. On December 29, 1170, with their swords in hand, they pursue Becket through Canterbury Cathedral. Some priests rush him to safety, until they arrive at the entrance to the sanctuary. Though his friends encourage him to continue running, here he stops, though the knights are just yards away. "I am not in danger: only near to death," he says,[2] and orders a priest who has bolted the cathedral door to open it, whereupon the knights kill him.

Throughout *Murder in the Cathedral*, T. S. Eliot's play of Becket's martyrdom, the archbishop is continually warned of the threat of death if he remains in Canterbury. But none should fear his possible death, he says, for "the hungry hawk / Will only soar and hover" until there is an "End" that will be "simple, sudden, God-given."[3] Thomas Becket, refusing to fear death, knows death is inevitable and believes

God will decide when it will be. As he tells the priests, "All things prepare the event."[4]

Martyrdom is an exceptional situation, so much so that most of us can admire it from afar, a noble example that is good for the theater but with little connection to our ordinary lives. Martyrs perceive something very few others do, an insight that gives them courage to face death. But if what the martyr understands is true, isn't it true for everyone born into a body and destined to die? Is it possible that being near to death but not in danger is for more than just the martyr? Saint Augustine, one of the most influential theologians and philosophers of Western culture, thought as much. He often preached at festivals of the martyrs. Rather than making them heroes of spectacular faith, in sermons dating back to AD 397 he deliberately made them "less dramatic, so as to stress the daily drama of God's workings"[5] in the lives of average people. Let us follow this direction and turn now to the spirit that animates the martyrs, looking for what it might mean for all of us "born of woman . . . of few days and full of trouble . . . [who] spring up like flowers and wither away; like fleeting shadows [who] do not endure" (Job 14:1–2).

The Event That Changes Everything

We have this idea in popular culture that once you see or hear or taste something of a unique nature, after the experience you will never be the same. Tritely, it may be a restaurant with the best lasagna, a computer game with the most stunning graphics, or audio speakers with great surround sound. More significantly, it may be a painting on the ceiling of the Sistine Chapel or a location like Victoria Falls or the Grand Canyon. Whatever it is, the implication is that you will never taste or see or hear the same again.

The resurrection of Jesus Christ from the dead was, for the first Christians, that kind of event. It was so radical an experience that at first they had difficulty accepting that it had actually happened. They had the writings of the Old Testament, which spoke of a Messiah who would suffer and die, yet afterward see "the light of life" (Isa. 53:11). They had heard Jesus speak repeatedly of his suffering, death, and resurrection in the three years he was with them.[6] Yet even after the event, knowing that the tomb where Jesus had been placed two days before was empty, they still had trouble recognizing that what Jesus had told them had come true. Only after he appeared to them, talked to them, and ate with them were they finally able to fathom the truth that Jesus was alive.[7]

And right away they realized that life would never be the same. From then on, everything had to be organized around that historically decisive event, and the most important thing was to be faithful witnesses to what they had seen and heard in the most straightforward terms possible.

> For what I received I passed on to you as of first importance, that Christ died for our sins according to the Scriptures, that he was buried, that he was raised on the third day according to the Scriptures, and that he appeared to Cephas, and then to the Twelve. After that, he appeared to more than five hundred of the brothers and sisters at same time, most of whom are still living, though some have fallen asleep. Then he appeared to James, then to all the apostles, and last of all he appeared to me also. (1 Cor. 15:3–8)

Tradition has it that many of the early followers of Jesus, including Paul who wrote these words, were martyred for their commitment to the resurrected Christ. But it didn't stop with those who had seen him; it lit a flame that passed on to succeeding generations. During the epidemics of plague and pestilence in the second and third centuries, when many were dying, most ran from the sick. The early Christians, "learning not to fear death,"[8] were willing to care for the victims, though many of them died as a result.[9] For the surrounding culture, "how they love one another" and "how they are ready even to die" were the most distinguishing characteristics of these early Christian communities.[10]

Once again we meet the spirit of the martyr who, having seen something, can never "unsee" it and now interprets everything through a completely new thought structure. Why was it "of first importance" that Jesus Christ suffered, died, was buried, and was resurrected on the third day? What changed about the way they perceived life and death that made them different people? What might it mean for others, even us, who perceive the same thing and who make a similar effort to diligently apply it to the way we live and the way we die? Let's look at some things offered by a view of life in which the climax of the story occurred in the first century, when Jesus Christ rose from the dead.

A New Plausibility Structure

When Paul wrote to the people at Corinth, he pointed to the death and resurrection of Jesus Christ from the dead as a matter of first importance, for one simple reason: if Christ was raised from the dead, then the same power that defeated death and raised him can also raise us from the dead (1 Cor. 15:20–22). Because they found the tomb empty, because the first followers of Jesus saw him alive and embodied, because Jesus later ascended into heaven and has promised to return again when all will be raised from the dead, then everything is different. Hidden here is what the martyrs know that gives them the strength to face death with courage. Here lies the reason we can live, knowing that death does not have the final answer. And here too lies the hope that we can pursue health and organize health care from outside the shadow of death. But to do that, we need to consider how this new plausibility structure differs from other options.

To ground this new structure correctly, we must see the distinction between resurrection and resuscitation. The teaching of the Christian church is not a return to this life; it is not a resuscitation of the dead, as if we were in an accident, our heart stopped beating, and someone got the paddles on us just in time and brought us back here. Being bound to our present kind of life forever and ever would more resemble hell than heaven, more like "making mud pies in a slum because he cannot imagine what is meant by the offer of a holiday at the sea. We are far too easily pleased."[11]

No, the resurrection promised is a new life in a new heaven and a new earth. God's good for us is not a continuation, a gradual improvement, or a maximization of the "good" of this life. It is completely different from the present, a new order where "the sound of weeping and of crying will be heard in it no more. Never again will there be in it an infant who lives but a few days; or an old man who does not live out his years. . . . No longer will they build houses and others live in them, or plant and others eat. . . . Nor will they bear children doomed to misfortune" (Isa. 65:19–23).[12] It is a radical new life far beyond any future we could construct or imagine.

Then there is the place of the body. As already noted, "rescuing the body," a troublesome issue for all ages, has been a particular challenge for modern Western culture with our increasing ability to manipulate and marginalize it. We previously spoke of the stunning revelation that God would "in-carnate," be with us in a body, showing us its importance for our life on earth. But in the climax of the story, he is raised from death in that same human body, marking its importance for the life to come. We are bodily beings now and will be so in eternity.[13] Once again the contrast is stark: rather than efforts to supersede the body, the body is an integral part of who we are and who we will be.[14]

With the climax of the story in the middle of history, a new order to come—completely different from the present one—and immortal life given rather than gotten, the narrative of the resurrection must of necessity clash with many other narratives that inform our thinking. The "coming of age" narrative of the Enlightenment promised worldwide progress through science, reason, and a benevolent civilized society; the narrative of the buffered self and self-authorization offers the hope of a safe personal world through control and choice; trans-humanist narratives will bring eternal life by connecting our minds to mechanics. In each case, life comes through avoiding death. But in the resurrection story new life can come only through death. The hold of other categories of thought is great, and the nature of the resurrection so original, that we may have trouble thinking through what this revelation means. Breaking the power of death by confronting and accepting death, central to the spirit of the martyr, is a paradox of the resurrection that we must explore further.

Destined to Die

The counterintuitive message of the resurrection is that the path to life is through death. Other narratives that would fulfill our desire for immortality by avoiding death leave the power of death unbroken and the fear of death intact. Only through the acceptance of death can death be defeated.

Throughout the Gospels and other writings of the New Testament, at the heart of the message is that Jesus was destined to die. Rather than a rejection of the frailty, fragility, and finitude of the human experience, Jesus lived with all of life's limitations. Over and over he reiterated that his was a life of dependence, and in dependence on God, he knew that he, the Son of God, was destined to die at an appointed time.[15] It was no accident that Jesus died. But neither was it a passive surrender to the power of death. Instead Jesus chose to accept his destiny, though he was tempted to reject it, even to the very end.[16]

Hanging on the cross with a short time left to live, he was repeatedly challenged to use his power to save himself, first by the people, then by the Roman soldiers, and finally by one of the criminals who was hanging on a cross next to him. You saved others, they said, so why not save yourself? (Luke 23:35–39). Despite possessing the power to do so, he remained dependent on God, and in his willingness to die he defeated death by dying and rising from the dead, becoming the source of life for all who would follow after him. Again we see the crucial importance of the resurrection: without it, Jesus lived a heroic life, but he is dead and in the grave, and his life has little applicability for us; but because of the resurrection, his life and willingness to die matter immensely for us, who likewise are destined to die.

Once the power of death is broken, like a dam that gives way, the pressure upon this life for immortality is released, opening the way for embracing life without rejecting our finite humanity. Dietrich Bonhoeffer, whose own life's engagement in resistance to the Nazi regime led to his execution by hanging when he was thirty-nine years old, both demonstrated by example and described in his writing this open embrace:

> Where, however, it is recognized that the power of death has been broken, where the miracle of the resurrection and new life shines right into the world of death, there one demands no eternities from life. One takes from life what it offers, not all or nothing, but good things and bad, important things and unimportant, joy and pain. One doesn't cling anxiously to life, neither does one throw it lightly away. One is content with measured time and does not attribute eternity to earthly things. One leaves to death the limited

right it still has, but one expects the new human being in the new world only from beyond death, from the power that has conquered death.[17]

Recognizing that our desire for transformation cannot be completed in history, we are no longer controlled by the fact that we are destined to die, nor do we expect that this life can give us all we need. When we don't "cling anxiously to life," we are freed to embrace it more fully.

A Healthy Love of Life

If we are no longer enslaved by our fear of death and, like the martyrs, have learned to face it, it might be thought that we would no longer care about this life. But the result is just the opposite. No longer demanding eternity from this life, we learn to love it for what it is, caring for it fully, cherishing it truly, and suffering with it honestly.

There is a moment in the life of Jesus that quietly illuminates this. It is a well-known event, only a few days before Jesus himself will die, when he learns that his friend Lazarus is deathly ill. Jesus knows the family well, having spent time in their home, and was particularly close to Lazarus's sisters, Mary and Martha. By the time he arrives, it has been four days since Lazarus died; he has already been laid in the tomb, and his sisters are in the throes of grief. The people standing around cannot understand why Jesus, who could open the eyes of the blind, didn't keep Lazarus from dying. But Jesus has a better plan: to raise him from the dead. Yet despite Jesus's understanding, exceeding anything we could ever know, that the power of the resurrection is greater than the power of death, in this profound moment he shares the sadness of those he loves and weeps with them (John 11:1–37).

Yes, the power of the resurrection frees us from the dominion of death. But sickness is still scary, aging difficult, suffering painful, and dying frightful. The separation of death will always be sad, and we will grieve the loss of each unique and irreplaceable person from our lives. Life remains precious outside the shadow of death and is not relinquished serenely as if unimportant. When offered, it is at great cost, as are all acts of deep love, because human life is valuable, and actions of self-giving, whether in small deeds or in full surrender, will always be hard. Thomas Becket, and those who gave their lives in the first century long ago, or Martin Luther King, Óscar Romero, and others who have given their lives more recently, did not accept death because they did not care about life. In fact they cared very much— which makes their sacrifice all the more honorable.

But the resurrection, as we already said, though it invites great heroism, also offers new ways to live for ordinary people, like you and me, in everyday circumstances. "God has many martyrs in secret," Augustine reminds us. "Sometimes you shiver with fever: you are fighting. You are in bed: it is you who are the athlete."[18] Listen to the story of one such athlete who ran the race well until the end.

Not a Martyr, but Still a Hero

John was a missionary in Africa for thirty-five years. He returned to the United States at age sixty-five but continued his commitment to Congo by returning every one or two years to support the projects and people he knew and loved. On one of his trips he began having lower abdominal pain. He consulted a local physician, who treated him for an intestinal infection, but his symptoms grew worse. When he began to see blood in his urine, he and his wife knew that they must return home.

John was soon diagnosed with bladder cancer. His primary care physician referred him to an oncologist, who explained the facts: most people will die within twelve months, but treatment can prolong life, maybe even cure it. Some family members were sure he would beat this cancer. But John and his wife had seen a lot during their years in Africa—they had come to know that life is risky and cancer treatment has no guarantees. Nevertheless, they were willing to try.

The next six months were a difficult time. John had many side effects from his treatment. He was frequently nauseated and unable to eat, at other times in bed or admitted to the hospital because of fever and possible infections. Though family was near, he was usually too ill to be with them. He rarely had the energy to meet with friends or write emails of support to his contacts around the world. When the news came back that the cancer had advanced despite treatment, he was offered another course of treatment, but now with much less chance of benefit.

John considered his situation, but with a different perspective from six months ago. He still listened to the numbers that told him of the probabilities of improvement and the list of side effects. He noted and appreciated the hopeful attitude of his doctor. But he knew his days were numbered and was thinking more about what he still hoped to do. His wife was not surprised when John told his doctor that he did not want further treatment. He decided to take a different risk, to live with the cancer and do as much as he could in the days that remained.

John lived for six more months, in much better health during most of that time than the previous six months. He died at home, surrounded by family and friends and supported by hospice. When I asked his wife afterward whether she thought they had made the right decisions, she said there were no regrets. They were glad they took the risk of treatment, hoping for cure if not good benefit, even though they were disappointed with the results. But they were also happy that they did not continue treatment. During the last few months of his life, John used what remaining health he had seeing friends in different parts of the United States and sharing many good times with family. He told his wife that he didn't think living for very long beyond his ability to give his life for others made much sense, and he had made it his final mission to tell as many people as possible how faithful God had been to him throughout his life. She said this sense of destiny and purpose gave him satisfaction that lasted to the end of his life.

Some wonder with good reason if it is "impossible for our technological culture ever to regain the naïve confidence in Destiny which had for so long been shown by simple men when dying."[19] The human ability to modify and manipulate the conditions of death, the uncertain line between life and death, and the absence of a common culture that accepts transcendence has clearly changed the parameters.[20] Yet John's story offers hope, as do many others. He retained faith in a charged world, specifically "charged with the grandeur of God."[21] John lived his life listening because he believed God was still speaking, and at the end he knew the time and how to use it well. He believed in the resurrection of Jesus Christ as the hope of God for this world. Within its overarching narrative, each of us is invited to understand our own story, know the time, and face death without fear.

Not Just for One Day but for Every Day

If we set aside until the end of our days what we know is true because of the resurrection, we make it like a living will: a good thing to have when the time comes but not very important until then. But the fear of death hovers over all of life. If we step out from beneath that shadow, the light cannot help but shine everywhere —especially if we recognize the darkness of our days without it.

Harvard theologian Arthur McGill, in his book *Death and Life: An American Theology*, does an excellent job of showing the pervasive influence of death in our modern life. He begins with a candid reminder from Augustine that "in fact, from the moment a man begins to exist in this body which is destined to die, he is involved all the time in a process whose end is death."[22] Simply stated, which of us is not nearer to death this year than we were last year? The problem, McGill says, is not this ongoing failure of life that ends with our death but our unwillingness to accept that we are dying daily. Instead, haunted every day by the fear of death, we make life a continual struggle to avoid need:

> So far as we reject living as a needy and hungry creature who is constantly given being by God, so far as we see our identity as wholly in terms of a reality which we can have and which we can securely label with our own name, we live under the dominion of death; we live under the dominion of dispossession. We live in terror of death, of having this bit of reality which we call ourselves, taken from us. Our whole existence is controlled by that terror.[23]

McGill's contention is straightforward though disturbing, particularly for the materialistic North American culture he is addressing: the power of death causes us to fear neediness as a regular experience of life. Integrating the terms we have used thus far into his argument, our desire for invulnerability and control is none other than death at work in our daily lives. Now we see the basis for our desire to possess, because the more we possess, the less we need. But defining ourselves by our possessions only reinforces death as the absolute enemy—death, as the final end of all having and possessing, will take away our identity by taking away our possessions. Living in a culture of death, we will do anything to avoid being in need.

Following his thesis through, when we are no longer bound by the power of death, we are freed from our demand for control and desire for invulnerability. Learning to rest in neediness, our release from the fear of death has immediate impact. First, grounded in a resurrection confidence that God will be reliable to nourish us daily, we learn to receive without demanding to possess. Second, no longer expecting that we can avoid need, we learn to give while still in need and do not require that our giving must supply all that is missing for our neighbor. We receive in need, and in our insufficiency we give, knowing that our giving will not remove the need of our neighbor. In common vulnerability, we learn to share.

If relief of neediness, either ours or our neighbors', is no longer expected or demanded, we have an opportunity to face in a fresh way the dilemma of a world where need always exceeds resources. As we turn to the issue of justice in health care, learning to share the world's goods from the perspective of common vulnerability has important implications.

Reimagining the
Good of Health

Just Community

Is There Enough?

You shall know the truth and the truth shall make you odd.

Flannery O'Connor

Flannery O'Connor was twenty-five years old when she was diagnosed with lupus, a disease named for the erosive facial rash that looks like the bite of a wolf. For the rest of her life she battled both the disease and the effects of cortisone used to treat it, eventually depending on crutches to get around. Late in life, when very ill, she wrote to a friend, "The wolf, I'm afraid, is inside tearing up the place."[1] One month later, at the age of thirty-nine, she was dead.

Though she minimized the impact of the disease on her life and writing, it was because of her illness that she was forced to return to her birthplace of Georgia and live her remaining years on a small farm. Only able to write for two or three useful hours a day before fatigue set in, her circumscribed life could have been a stifling limitation. Instead, it became a great strength. Accepting these limitations as factors that sharpened her view of reality, she saw odd but universal truths from the particularities of her place and became one of the most influential American novelists of the twentieth century. "We are limited human beings," she said, "and the novel is a product of our best limitations."[2]

During her life, Flannery O'Connor apprehended the "unseen" by immersing herself in the "seen" of her rural Southern culture, expressing her strange but insightful view of reality in her writing. Many like me, immersed in medicine at the margins with the disenfranchised, have also apprehended some strange and often unseen truths. If they make us odd, they can also give us vision and the depth to endure in striving for justice in health care. Succinctly stated, they are: (1) seeing *you* depends on seeing *me* in you; (2) my health depends on your health; and (3) the health of society depends on how it cares for its poorest members. Whether odd to you or obvious, each of these dependencies needs a closer look.

We Are All Vulnerable

Like Humpty Dumpty long ago, we have deeply desired a stance of invulnerability from which to pursue health. Yet the disturbing truth that we are vulnerable and needy remains firmly fixed at the center of our being. This recognition may yet be the source of our redemption. But it can also lead us to work for justice, especially when we realize that we share this vulnerability to suffering and death with every other human being. To explain, let's look at a natural reaction, a recent event, and a mysterious reality that, though we see it, and then see it again, we still have trouble understanding what we saw.

A Common Experience

When I met Walter, I knew it was something bad. He was my age but looked like he had been ill for many months; thin and wasted, he was holding his stomach and writhing in pain on the exam table. He was living on the streets, which was common for patients who came to this health center for the homeless, but few would have waited this long to see a doctor. "Please help me," he said, and I felt a deep desire to do so.

It is a common experience in the doctor-patient relationship to identify with certain patients because we see ourselves in them. We may have a comparable family life, perhaps with an absent parent; or a patient miscarries, causing us to remember our own miscarriage; or, like Flannery O'Connor, our patient has lupus, just like our sister. When I considered the possibility that my patient might have undiagnosed colon cancer, it was not an objective hypothesis but a subjective fear. Identifying with him by our same age, I personally felt his vulnerability to it.

We worked as a staff beyond the usual, getting him to the emergency room, helping him with follow-up appointments, and arranging for aftercare when the hospital discharged him after his operation—for colon cancer. I knew all along that my actions were focused by the awareness that he could be me. Was it influencing me too much? Or did I worry that in other cases I wouldn't be as committed and caring, because I wouldn't see myself in the next patient as I did when I looked at Walter?

A Recent Epidemic

The ability to see ourselves in others is an odd gift. By it, perhaps more than anything else, our hearts are enlarged and our compassion aroused. But then we must act, doing what we can to help the hurting person. To permit the pain of another to come near because we know that we are likewise vulnerable is also a burden—but better to be burdened than buffered and blind.

Many will recall the most recent outbreak of the Ebola virus that began in December 2013. It was not until August 2014 that the World Health Organization declared it a "Public Health Emergency of International Concern" (PHEIC),[3] followed by a resolution by the United Nations Security Council in September 2014 establishing the UN Mission for Ebola Emergency Response, a resolution with more support than any since the founding of the United Nations in 1946. It was a strong response but late, coming many months into an outbreak that had already unnecessarily claimed many lives and become one of the most devastating health crises of the twenty-first century.[4] Localized to three West African countries with limited health care systems,[5] early availability of simple medical care and basic resources such as protective gowns, gloves, and intravenous fluids could have significantly reduced the spread of the disease and high fatality rate.

But for many, the problems of Africa are not our problems, because, as poet Rudyard Kipling observed, "all the people like us are we, and everyone else is they."[6] Disengaged from the mothers and fathers who were losing their children or the children who were losing their parents, the Ebola crisis was a problem of "them," not "us."

Yet the reality is that pathogens cross borders even if our care does not—which leads only to greater separation and higher walls. Fearing the possibility that Ebola would come to their own country, many called for quarantine of the affected countries with restriction of all travel in and out. Those who volunteered to go and help, rather than being seen as heroes, were vilified as dangerous risk takers who would carry the virus home and infect their communities.

As in days past, the arrival of contagious epidemics tests the heart at the same time that it challenges protocols for containment. The latest Ebola epidemic was far worse than any prior outbreak. But it will not be the last. To respond wisely and kindly to the next global epidemic, or to unjust systems that oppress many, or even the needs of one single neighbor, we need a sense of shared vulnerability.[7] When we live as if we are invulnerable, every threat frightens us, making our desire for control greater and our need to separate ourselves stronger. But when we acknowledge our common condition, it opens our hearts to care. Sharing the vulnerability of life with others may even help us perceive a mystery that the usual senses would normally miss.

Twice You Have Seen It, Yet Still You Don't Understand?

Most people familiar with the Bible know there are four Gospels. Written by different authors, each one offers a unique window through which to view the life of Jesus Christ. Sometimes they report the same incident; then there are events that appear only in one Gospel. But no event is repeated as often as the feeding of thousands with only a few bits of food. Each author saw its importance and placed it in his Gospel. But Matthew and Mark report it twice, since it happened on two different occasions. Given how much they had to leave out, why would they choose to include two events with such similar circumstances?

In both instances thousands of people travel to a remote place to find Jesus. There he teaches them many things, heals the sick, and restores the lame and the blind. After many hours pass, the people are hungry, but food is scarce, and they are far from town. In each case, Jesus responds in a similar way. He asks them what they have: one time there are five thousand to feed with five loaves of bread and two fish; the next time four thousand have gathered, with seven loaves but no fish. Then Jesus gives thanks for the food, breaks it into pieces, and distributes it to everyone. And after all are satisfied, there are basketfuls of leftovers.[8]

Immediately after, Jesus gets into a boat to go to the other side of the lake with those who helped him distribute the food. Jesus wants to teach them something and uses the analogy of yeast. But his friends don't get it—they are worried that they have only one loaf of bread with them, and they think he is talking about real food. "Why are you talking about having no bread?" Jesus asks them. "Do you still not see or understand? Are your hearts hardened? Do you have eyes but fail to see, and ears but fail to hear? And don't you remember? When I broke the five loaves for the five thousand, how many basketfuls of pieces did you pick up?" Twelve, they remembered. "And when I broke the seven loaves for the four thousand, how many basketfuls of pieces did you pick up?" Seven, they remembered. And Jesus asks again, "Do you still not understand?" (Mark 8:14–21).

As long as we are trapped in a myth of scarcity, we will struggle with the mystery of abundance. Living as if we can be invulnerable, we take every step to avoid need. But there is never enough in that world. Forced to close our eyes to the suffering of others, we accept the rules of a zero-sum game. It is a competitive game, with only winners and losers, a division, as Wendell Berry reminds us, harsher than "the other social divisions: that of the more able and the less able, or that of the richer and the poorer, or even that of the rulers and the ruled. These latter divisions have existed throughout history and at times, at least, have been ameliorated by social and religious ideals that instructed the strong to help the weak."[9] But when my sufficiency depends on your insufficiency, because of how little there is to go around, then, like the conversation in the boat, we will fail to understand, close our eyes to the needs of the world, and never see the possibility for abundance. Which bring us to another odd truth about the deep connection between my life and your life.

Health Is a Communal Event

Most modern political and economic thought and action prioritize private and personal goals over communal care and the common good. Our current health care spending, predicated on individual fear and worry, creates more and more services with less and less value. Several studies have documented that in communities where there are more doctors and more hospital beds, though more money is spent on health care, the outcomes are not better;[10] paradoxically, in some analyses, the outcomes are worse.[11] At the same time, our growth in spending does not correlate with increased care for those who need it most. Though one of every five dollars for health care in the world is spent in the United States, one in every eight people is uninsured,[12] most of them poorer and sicker than the general population and with little access to care beyond the emergency room.

The individual pursuit of health contorts the role of medicine, asking it to deliver us from our finitude, our mortality, and our human vulnerability to suffering. But instead of good health care and better health, the end result is too much health care for some, too little health care for others, and less health for all. We have multiplied the means of health care without a good understanding of the proper end of health, resulting in increased waste and greater injustice.

Though his subject is economic theory and practice, author John Medaille illustrates the confusion between means and ends with an anecdote from his youth that has application to our subject. When he was a boy living in New York City, very few people had cars. But fifteen cents bought a subway token and access to some of the most diverse cultural and recreational experiences in the world. Means were scarce, since few individuals had cars, but transportation was abundant for these seven-year-old children who could reach anywhere in New York on the subway. Fast-forward to his adult life in an affluent suburb, where many families had more than one car, but his children had very little transportation. They could not go anywhere unless someone took them. The scarce means but abundant transportation of the subway was replaced by abundant cars but scarce transportation, with children restricted to when their parents could find time to take them.[13]

Medaille argues that a proper economy of resources should provide for a relative abundance of ends using relatively scarce means. When we reverse the terms, we replace "robust systems designed according to some notion of the common good" into "narrow systems designed on the premises of individualism." We multiply our means, whether it is cars or health care, at great expense but make the ends, be they transportation or health, problematic. We lack "a vision of the common good, and a proper distribution function informed by that vision."[14]

The notion of the common good has particular relevance for the formation of good health care because of the critical connection between communal health and individual health. In fact, individual health may even be a misnomer, as Berry suggests:

> I believe that the community—in the fullest sense: a place and all its creatures—is the smallest unit of health and that to speak of the health of an isolated individual is a contradiction in terms.[15]

Building on our awareness of shared vulnerability, let's consider some reasons why we can only be as healthy as our neighbor.

We have already made mention of communicable diseases. Besides Ebola, which is not particularly dangerous apart from direct contact, when we speak of diseases transmitted through the air, like influenza, or by means of a common vector like the mosquito, as is the case with malaria, the health of my neighbor is immediately important to my health. If they are ill with the disease, then I am at risk; the better their health, and the sooner they receive care, the better for me and the entire community.

Loneliness is not communicable, but it too can diminish the health of a community. When sad people drink to numb the pain, they hurt only themselves. But if one of them gets behind a wheel, drives drunk, and hits a child in the street, the whole community suffers.

The broad effects of violence on the health of a community deepen the relationship even further. Although the greatest violence is concentrated in the most disadvantaged communities, and those who perpetrate the violence are most often its victims,[16] fear of crime and violence percolates throughout the whole neighborhood and beyond, increasing anxiety and putting everyone on edge. This hypervigilance affects quality of life in general, reducing trust in neighbor, increasing a sense of helplessness, and making us all nervous to go out at night or even feel safe in our own home. Constant hyperarousal also has direct detrimental effects on physical health; for example, the much greater burden of heart disease in unsafe neighborhoods has been related to exposure to chronic and acute stress.[17] Thus any efforts to reduce violence, whether we support law enforcement to reduce current violence, or improve educational opportunities and strengthen families to prevent future violence, are beneficial to the health of all.

More generally, when violence in a community is generated out of the hopelessness and anger of those who feel left behind as society progresses around them, it should encourage our desire for a fairer distribution of societal goods that lifts up all communities. Epidemiologists Wilkinson and Pickett, in their book *The Spirit Level*, carry this argument into multiple areas of health. Looking at numerous associations between income inequality and health, including teen pregnancy, mental illness, and obesity, they conclude that what matters in determining health is less the overall wealth of that society, assuming a certain basic level,[18] and more how well that society reduces inequalities in wealth.[19] Pertinent to our discussion, the better health found in societies that have a more even distribution of wealth not only benefits the poor but also every other sector of society, including the rich.[20]

So it matters to avoid extreme disparities in wealth because they contribute to disparities in health. Or as John Calvin was reported to have said, "Wealth is like manure; it works best when it is spread, but stinks when it is in one big pile." Whether health or wealth, the analogy has useful contributions to make to the broader social and political discussion.[21] But what we must not miss, as individuals rightly concerned for our personal health, is the value of community health for everyone's health, both rich and poor, and everyone in between.

When we see the pursuit of health as a communal activity to our own benefit, we will more readily place the common good at the center, and accept more scarce means for the sake of more abundant ends.

The Preferential Option for the Poor Who Are Sick

Our final truth may be the oddest of all. To prove that the health of a society depends on how it cares for its poorest members would need a measuring stick that none of us possesses. But the care of "the least of these," with careful attention to how our actions affect the poorest of our neighbors, may be the most important thing we do for our health.

Maria was forty-two years old when she came to the health center as a new patient. She first noticed a lump in her breast six months earlier and since then had been trying to find a clinic that would see her. But because she had no insurance, she was turned down or told there was a waiting list of many months. Because of our health center's well-worn connections to charitable services, she was soon diagnosed with breast cancer, but by then it had spread to other organs. Maria received two years of chemotherapy, which extended her life but could not save it. She was forty-four years old when she died, leaving behind her husband and two teenage children.

We cannot know if Maria would have lived longer if she had found access to health care sooner. But at the same time that she needed immediate care for breast cancer and could not find it, our society was spending nearly $8 billion per year screening for breast cancer in healthy, low-risk women.[22] At what ages and how often we screen for breast cancer, and the limits of its value, is a highly controversial subject.[23] But until we ensure that those with breast cancer, especially the poor among us, have access to care, it will have minimal impact on the health of our society. In the end we will be evaluated, as shepherds of our society's resources, not by whether we did everything we could but by whether we did everything we should for those who needed health care most.

If there is one theme in the Old Testament that cannot be missed, it is the call for justice and concern for the oppressed. From the moment God hears the cries of his people and delivers them from slavery in Egypt, the stage upon which faithful living will be judged has been set. Every society formed by God's people thereafter is expected to remember their enslavement as outsiders in Egypt and take special care of the weak, the poor, and the oppressed.[24] But over and over they act unjustly, though prophet after prophet warns them.[25] Finally, after repeated failures to keep the covenant, the people are sent into exile in Babylon. Here the word of God comes to them through the prophet Ezekiel:

> This is what the Sovereign LORD says: Woe to you shepherds of Israel who only take care of yourselves! Should not shepherds take care of the flock? . . . You have not strengthened the weak or healed the sick or bound up the injured. You have not brought back the strays or searched for the lost. (Ezek. 34:2, 4)

Because the shepherds have fattened themselves and left the sheep scattered and vulnerable, in one dramatic action God demotes them to sheep and takes their place as shepherd:

> For this is what the Sovereign LORD says: I myself will search for my sheep and look after them. . . . . I will bind up the injured and strengthen the weak, but the sleek and the strong I will destroy. . . . I myself will judge between the fat sheep and the lean sheep. Because you shove with flank and shoulder, butting all the weak sheep with your horns until you have driven them away, I will save my flock, and they will no longer be plundered. (Ezek. 34:11, 16, 20–22)

Six hundred years later, Jesus Christ, the Good Shepherd, would come to fulfill all that Ezekiel had promised the shepherd would do.[26]

An Opportunity and a Responsibility

And now we who follow after in the light and life of Jesus Christ are expected to act with the same heart of concern for the weak, the injured, and the stray. If instead we neglect them, we are like the shepherds of Israel who cared only for themselves, or like fat sheep who, already heavily laden with health care, push aside the weak and sick so that we can have more.

Though the challenge is great, we are comforted to know that we are called to care, not complete the task. Never expected to be God, we are only asked to do good so that the least among us with the greatest needs have access to the most care. In so doing, we prepare the way for what is to come:

> Prepare the way for the Lord, make straight paths for him. Every valley shall be filled in, every mountain and hill made low. The crooked roads shall become straight, the rough ways smooth. And all people will see God's salvation. (Luke 3:4–6, quoting Isa. 40:3–5)

We are strengthened to work with diligence and perseverance now because we know the salvation of God will one day bring full justice for all. Our penultimate actions here will not determine the ultimate justice that is to come.[27] But our actions now, prompted by an inner faith in what will be, have significant outward effects, as Dietrich Bonhoeffer reminds us:

> And this preparation is not only an inward process, but a visible creative activity on the greatest scale. "Every valley shall be lifted up." What has been pushed into the depths of human misery, what is lowly and humiliated, will be raised. There is a depth of human bondage, of human poverty, and of human ignorance that hinders the gracious coming of Christ. "Every mountain and hill shall be made low." If Christ is to come, all that is proud and high must bow. There is a degree of power, of wealth, and of knowledge that is a hindrance to Christ.[28]

Our choices make a difference. When we are motivated by fear and self-absorption, there will be extreme disparity and much injustice, deepening the distance between what is high and what is low. But when we see the bonds of our shared vulnerability, and if we work to reduce the disparities that separate us, we smooth the way for the coming of Christ.

It will never be easy to choose for the protection of the poorest and weakest in health care. The truth that their health matters to our health is indeed a strange one. Not only for us but for every generation, it has been difficult to take notice of Lazarus at the gate.[29] For one man who took sick while caring for others, it was a visitation in a dream that made him realize how much the cries of the poor matter.

It was Philadelphia in 1780, and "breakbone fever," an outbreak of dengue, was rapidly spreading through the city. Benjamin Rush, the only physician-signer of the Declaration of Independence and one of the most important physicians in the history of American medicine up to the Civil War, came down with the disease. One night, in the midst of his illness, he had a dream:

> A poor woman came to me just as I was getting into my chair in Penn Street, and begged me to visit her husband. I told her hastily, that I was worn out in attending poor people, and requested her to apply to another doctor.
>
> "Oh sir," she said, lifting up her hands, "you don't know how much you owe to your poor patients. It was decreed that you should die by the fever which lately attacked you, but the prayers of your poor patients ascended to heaven on your behalf, and your life is prolonged only on their account."[30]

He awoke in tears. As a scientific man, he seldom considered dreams as more than reactions to physical changes. Yet, he said, this dream "left a deep and lasting impression upon my mind. It increased my disposition to attend the poor and never, when I could serve them, to treat them in an uncivil manner."[31] Six years later Dr. Rush founded the Philadelphia Dispensary, the first clinic in the United States dedicated to quality care for the poor.

Once he understood, Dr. Rush never forgot the odd truth he learned that night in his dream. Can we be likewise moved by the odd truths of life that connect our lives to others? Left with a "deep and lasting impression upon our minds" that the manner in which we treat our neighbor, and particularly the weakest amongst us, has eternal significance, we too will desire to do our part for the sake of justice in health care.

10

The Cooperation of Faith and Medicine

The Hope for Salvation in the Midst of Pursuing Health

Consequently, we must take great care to employ the medical art, if it should be necessary, not as making it wholly accountable for our state of health or illness, but as redounding to the glory of God.

Basil, Bishop of Cappadocia, fourth century AD

A professor was asking a young friend in Mexico about his doctoral thesis. Juanito respectfully showed it to him, especially proud because he had dedicated it to the professor for all that he had learned from him. Always intrigued with what his professor was working on, he then asked him, *"Maestro, y qué tú haces ahora?"* (What are you up to now, professor?) *"Me ocupo de salud,"* he answered. (I've been thinking about health.) "Ah," the young man said, "very interesting, you have returned to theology."[1]

Why the Confusion?

An understandable misunderstanding—though for most people today the Spanish word *salud* means "health," Juanito was thinking of "salvation" because, in the older use of the language, it can mean salvation for the soul as easily as it can mean the physical health and well-being of the body. No wonder the confusion between health, usually seen as the focus of medicine, and salvation, typically understood as the domain of religion. In search of cooperation between faith and medicine,[2] we have a twofold task. First, as our story shows, the divide between health and salvation, bodily health and spiritual health, is a line much thinner than we who have been raised in the dualism of our age might think. Thus far in our discussion, we have tried to reduce that divide, showing the importance of our creation as embodied souls, and the reality of a material world still charged with mystery and the agency of God. Letting that divide enter into our hope for healing, we have driven faith and medicine apart, which has been alienating for the former and degrading for the latter. If we can reform the bonds that connect them, each will be the better for it.

But if the two are to cooperate well, we must do more than simply pull down the walls of separation and push them together into one indistinct whole. For the good of medicine and the value of faith, we must understand the different roles that each has to play. We will start by addressing a common misconception, that faith and science, as if oil and water, cannot mix. Then, in honest evaluation, we ask each side to admit their part in the problem. After acknowledging these failures and faults, we can more firmly offer some of the specific contributions that each has to make to healing. Finally we will look at what can happen when the two work together for a common purpose.

Why the Conflict?

The myth that science and faith are by nature incompatible finds its roots at the beginning of the modern era, when science was posed as the source of universal and provable truth, isolating religion to individual belief that was mostly superstitious.[3] This negative view of religion reinforced the need to see science and reason as separate from faith and religion, and, if truth be told, superior to it. But to see the true relation between faith and science, we must distinguish between science as a method of inquiry and science as ideology. The former flourishes in the context of faith, while the latter can function only on the basis of unscientific claims. This distinction is important to explain.

The origin and development of modern science in the sixteenth and seventeenth centuries took place at a time when Western culture held to a particular religious view of the world. As missionary and theologian Lesslie Newbigin describes the necessary precondition for the birth of science as we know it:

> It has been very plausibly argued that the decisive factor is to be found in the biblical vision of the world as both rational and contingent. For to put it briefly, if the world is not rational, science is not possible; if the world is not contingent, science is not necessary.[4]

Without a passionate faith in rational order, science as a method of inquiry would falter, stagnate, and die. But without a contingent world, all is fixed and immutable, making efforts to understand and improve it meaningless. Only because God has created a rational world will our investigations reveal repeatable patterns. And only because God has created a world with a measure of autonomy and contingency can we find the freedom to search, to experiment, and to learn for ourselves how things really are and what we can do to make them better.

On the other hand, when we expand beyond science as a method of inquiry and assume it to be the royal road to all knowledge, we make two unscientific claims about it: that "it will eventually know everything, and it will eventually solve all human problems."[5] This act of faith confuses theory with knowledge and infuses science with mystical powers, rightly understood only by an elite few who know everything or believe they soon will. Or as Walter Percy, a physician turned novelist, explains it:

Scientism is characterized less by the practice of a method of discovery and knowing than what can only be called a surrender of sovereignty and a willingness to believe almost as a matter of course that the scientific method by virtue of its spectacular triumphs and the near magic of its technology can be extrapolated to a quasi-religious all-construing worldview.[6]

Call it scientism, or call it pseudoscience, but as an all-pervading ideology, it is not the true science that God has gifted to all.

In fact, science and medicine have every reason to cooperate with faith and religion, in particular with that brand of faith that sees a world worth investigating because it has order that is discoverable. While this faith admires the scientific method for its ability to investigate and know, this union also accepts that the world is not fully knowable. In the cooperation of faith and medicine, knowledge that is empirically knowable is not threatened by knowledge that cannot be explained. Aware of knowledge that is unprovable but still valid, good medicine continues to value sound science but also appreciates mystery.

Medicine Must Acknowledge Its Limits

Many years ago, as I was preparing to go to Africa as a missionary physician, I heard a story about a physician who founded a hospital in Africa in the early 1900s. When he first arrived, the tools of medicine that he brought were meager in comparison to current standards, having only a few medicines and the ability to perform some simple operations. Yet he saw great power for healing in the methods he possessed. What caught my attention then, and still remember now, was his awareness of both the capabilities and the limits of medicine.

Early on, he realized that the cause of illness is bigger than medicine. So he decided to expand the possibilities for healing by cooperating with others in the community who were already recognized as sources of care and understanding. He sat with them and discussed some of the "patient" problems he was seeing, talking to them like colleagues with whom he was discussing "cases." Some of the problems were treatable with medical techniques—he taught them to recognize a patient with a strangulated hernia or a fever that was likely malaria, and he encouraged them to refer these patients to the hospital where he could operate or give quinine. But some of the problems had roots in contexts that needed cultural and social interpretations if they were to be understood and treated. He asked if he could refer some of his patients to them. And for things that were in between, where his medical care was useful but limited and the patient still suffered, he asked if they could work together. He believed in the good of medicine but also saw its boundaries and the need for a larger view that invited cooperation.

Regardless of how much more medicine can do now than then, medicine still has limits, and cooperation is still a good idea. But given its stupendous advances, medicine has overflowed its borders and assumed the role of savior from disease and death. Or has society, fueled by the utopian presumption that illness can be cured and death tamed, placed on medicine the impossible task of bandaging all of its wounds? Truly it is both. Modern medicine as well as the community that supports it have become confused about its purpose and transferred hope for salvation from the halls of faith to the corridors of medicine. But medicine cannot sustain this arrogant undertaking without becoming further corrupted. For the good of medicine and our own wise pursuit of health, we must help medicine to understand its proper role.

The Church Must Confess Its Failure

As a medical practitioner, I acknowledge the conceit of medicine as my own and share in its faults. Likewise, I am a member of the church, which has often been criticized for substituting institutional power for Christian love, and control and success for faith and trust.[7] I do not wish to avoid this judgment, nor do I assume that it is always true. But in lieu of rattling all the skeletons in this closet, and how overwhelming it would be if they all came out, we will confine ourselves to two related ways the church has failed in its interactions with the world of medicine.

First, the blunt truth is that today's church accepts far too passive a role in health care. Inhibited by the power and prestige of medicine, the church has often retreated into the small spaces that medicine permits it for a brief visit or a quiet prayer. With the miraculous technology that surrounds the patient in most medical settings, pastors, priests, and chaplains can feel small and insignificant before the people in white coats who seem to know so much more about the present condition and future prognosis. Just like rituals in other sacred spaces, those who come must bow before the doctor, genuflect at the nurses' station, dip their hands in the "holy water" dispensers on the wall, put on the appropriate robes and masks before seeing the patient in isolation, and, above all, be sure to depart before visiting hours are over.

But the church has no reason to cower. For the church knows the future in the light of God's promises, sees the possibility for healing from the most unexpected places, and holds a view of the sick as members of a community who, by being loved and loving others, still have important roles to play despite being infirm and in bed. If medicine is to be used wisely and the sick are to be restored to health, the church must step out of the shadows and bear witness to what it knows.

Second, rather than confronting the conceit found in medicine, the church often plays by the same rules, looking for its own tools and techniques to control the circumstances of health and sickness. Prayer, the sacraments, and other practices of the church have an important role to play in healing. But their primary function as invitations to God's presence and purpose is too often reduced to just another tool or technique to guarantee an outcome or control what God will do— especially when nothing else is working.

Let a biblical example illustrate the ease with which the people of God replace the actions of God with controllable forms of power. In the Old Testament there is a story of healing associated with an important symbol.[8] The people of God, on their way to the Promised Land, are in the middle of the desert. At the moment, they are in crisis because they are being bitten by venomous snakes. As many are dying, they go to Moses, their leader, and plead for relief. After speaking to God on behalf of the people, Moses is told to make a snake out of bronze and put it at the end of a pole, whereupon any who are bitten and look upon the bronze snake are healed. It is a miraculous event, and the people move on (Num. 21:4–9). But it is not the end of the snake.

Six hundred years later the bronze snake shows up again. Rather than accepting it as the uncontrollable means through which healing occurred once, the people have kept what Moses made and turned it into an item of worship (2 Kings 18:4). Presumably, the people believed in its ongoing power to heal, so a man-made object with no power apart from God has become an idol to which the people give devotion. How easily we substitute human constructs that seem to offer power and control for God, whose power we cannot control. Thus the prophet warns: "I will pronounce my judgments on my people because of their wickedness in forsaking me, in burning incense to other gods and in worshiping what their hands have made" (Jer. 1:16). Whether church or medicine, when we let our techniques—what our hands have made—take the place of God, it will cause us great confusion and a good deal of trouble.

Rather than seeking to substitute for God when he seems absent or ineffective,[9] or seeing him as merely a supplement to fill in the gaps when medicine fails, the church has the powerful ability to recognize the presence of God in the midst of uncertainty. In particular, the church knows that times of sickness and vulnerability may be the solemn occasion of God's unique visitation in a person's life, as John Donne's faithful prayer during sickness beautifully demonstrates:

> Eternal and most glorious God. . . . Thou alone dost steer my boat through all its voyage, but has a more especial care of it, when it comes to a narrow current, or to a dangerous fall of waters. Thou has a care of the preservation of my body in all the ways of my life; but, in the straits of death, open Thine eyes wider, and enlarge Thy Providence towards me so far that no illness or agony may shake and benumb the soul. . . . Do Thou so make my bed in all my sickness that, being used to Thy hand, I may be content with any bed of Thy making.[10]

Having faced the truth about limits and failures, we are in a better position to look at some specific ways that medicine and the church can contribute to a wise pursuit of health and a sound practice of medicine. These are not meant to be a comprehensive list or a new set of rules but opportunities and challenges. As each strives to fulfill its unique role, the good of health for all will grow as they work together toward a common purpose.

Contributions of Medicine

No one can better train caregivers in the proper method of inquiry and investigation than the science of medicine. The study of medicine will develop the curious mind that will always be looking for greater knowledge but never compromising high standards for scientific truth. This latter requirement will protect the patient from unproven theories and respect the divide between random or weak associations and probable cause-and-effect relationships. Knowing the strength of the findings and applying them in the context of a particular patient, medicine can offer what will most likely benefit and avoid what is unnecessary and wasteful. While a cholesterol pill daily for Mr. Jones may be beneficial, for Mr. Smith it is unlikely to make a difference.

Though the church can help, medicine is in a unique position to use the numerous situations its practitioners face as training for how to be present with those in pain. Those in the profession will use all their skills to alleviate the pain of illness to the fullest extent possible. Yet while seeking to relieve avoidable pain, medicine will accept suffering as a part of the human experience and be committed to never abandon the sufferer. Many have been taught only the first half of the equation, leaving patients fearful that when cure is no longer possible, their doctor will no longer see them. But many a good practitioner has committed to staying with patients long after treatments have ceased to work. As one friend experienced it: "I gain so much walking with my dying patients on their final journey."

Medicine can also help people to learn to live in and through their bodies, teaching the limits of the body and the wisdom that comes from accepting those limits. Aging will not be seen as a disorder to be corrected but as a time of adjustment for continued growth as we face increasing limitations as part and parcel of our being embodied living creatures. Likewise, the restrictions of imperfect bodies will not be viewed as automatic barriers to full life but as possible means through which life is found—and sometimes taught only by those who are living it. As one father said when taking his daughter with spina bifida to a father-daughter dance, "It's harder for me . . . than it is for Michelle. She has a blast! I look around and say, 'What a tragedy that she can't do that.' She says, 'Come on, let's dance, Dad.'"[11] Helping people to dance should be one of the good purposes of medicine.

Medicine, knowing much about the world of disease, can bridge the world of illness with the world of health, using wisdom gained helping the sick to teach the healthy what they can do to protect health. In one short hour a doctor may leave the hospital where a patient has kidney failure caused by diabetes and is on dialysis, only to see another patient in the office who has diabetes that is poorly controlled but not yet with advanced complications. Vividly seeing these connections, medicine can help the still well to see the value of good care of their body for staying well. Medicine will not portray such good care as a guarantee of health but as sound advice for healthy behaviors that respect the body.

Medicine can help those who are ill to move from the fearful unknown to the more fully known. Though the exact outcome can never be known for any patient, the profession's understanding of what a patient has and what often happens will mitigate the patient's fear and draw him out of isolation into the context of human care. Sometimes, it is as simple as giving it a name. For example, when I first arrived in Africa, the early months were difficult. By the third month, I was tired all the time and had little appetite or energy. Was it the heat? Was it the stress? Was I depressed? Then one day my urine changed color. I went to a doctor, who diagnosed hepatitis A. Though I knew the next two months of sickness would be little affected by any treatment, just knowing what I had and what would likely happen was a great relief. Just by understanding what is happening and will likely happen, medicine can help even if it cannot cure.

Medicine can actively invite family, friends, and church into the medical context rather than marginalizing them. Knowing that health is connected to community, medicine will invite this involvement and learn more about what the patient needs from who the patient is, which only those who know and love the patient can provide.

Finally, medicine should sustain both a strong commitment to the individual and a public responsibility to society. Therefore, in balancing the needs of individual patients with what is good for the health of society, it will focus its greatest resources on those with the greatest need. If having mammograms for the many means restricted access for those with breast cancer, or if high-cost infertility treatments for some is accompanied by the absence of good prenatal care for others, medicine will ensure that limited resources are engaged for the most important priorities.

Contributions of the Church

The church uniquely grasps the concept of covenant, because it is the core of a relationship with God. With promise and fidelity as the foundations of this covenant, the church has an important role to play in reminding medicine of its best traditions—the doctor-patient relationship thrives as a covenant of trust but atrophies as a contract for purchased services. Reinforcing the practitioner's commitment to this essential relationship, patients will find a trustworthy place to go when ill or in fear of sickness.[12]

The church has a strong understanding of indebtedness and grace. Thus it can remind health care professionals of the debt they owe their patients for the skill and art they possess. All who have learned about the body were taught through the offer of another's body. Beginning with those who donate their body for dissection to teach anatomy, to the patients who submit their body in sickness and health for examination, medicine learns from its patients. It is often the poor whose bodies teach the newest doctors and nurses, and every patient afterward continues to instruct if we in the profession remain willing to learn. Health care professionals who care as if in debt to their patients and community will always care more humbly, justly, and wisely.

The church also has a deep understanding of forgiveness. The medical community is growing in its understanding of the role of guilt in disease. Too often, even though we can fix the body, the patient's illness continues as a consequence of unresolved guilt and shame. The church can help to heal patients through the acknowledgment of guilt and the release of shame through forgiveness. A passage in the book of James addresses this: "Is anyone among you sick? Let them call the elders of the church to pray over them and anoint them with oil in the name of the Lord. And the prayer offered in faith will *make* the sick person *well*; the Lord will *raise* them *up*. If they have sinned, they will be forgiven" (James 5:14–15). In the midst of a safe and caring church community, the person can be "made well" (*sōzō*, a Greek word that also means "salvation") and "raised up" (*egeirō*, the same Greek word applied to Jesus's release from the grave), even if the medical outcome is limited or the cure of the particular disease impossible.

The church understands that we are on pilgrimage in a world that is not all there is. A fatal mistake in pursuing health and practicing medicine is thinking we have no destiny beyond this world. Although the church herself at times struggles to remember, no other institution is better able to remind us that hope does not lie in the nostalgia of the past, the realities of the present, or the certainties of a calculated future. Such a reminder will place our desire for health in the context of our higher purpose, helping us to use medicine well in service to our noble call.

The fact that we suffer, and have a God who allows it, remains one of the greatest threats to an ordered, impersonal universe of solvable problems. Rather than seeking to explain it or control it, the church can dwell in suffering without recoil, because, in communion with a personal and present God who suffered with us, it believes in a redemptive promise that absorbs suffering.

In Psalm 84 the themes of pilgrimage and redemptive suffering are brought together: "Blessed are those whose strength is in you, whose hearts are set on pilgrimage. As they pass through the Valley of Baka, they make it a place of springs" (vv. 5–6). The valley of Baka, from the Hebrew word meaning "to weep," is a valley of tears. On our journeys through life, we will all pass through this valley; those whose journey is marked by dependence on God's strength can transform those tears into springs of life-giving water. In a world of sickness that regularly encounters suffering and tragedy that it cannot explain, the church's awareness of this great mystery can be a source of strength for both practitioner and patient.

Finally, the church understands that in the economy of God, "the one who gathered much did not have too much, and the one who gathered little did not have too little. Everyone had gathered just as much as they needed" (Ex. 16:18). The church can regularly remind medicine and society of these principles of distribution for health care and advocate for the protection of the most vulnerable when these principles are neglected. [13]

And at the end of it all, when the world seems oblivious to what the church is saying, then let it show what it means by what it does.

A Model of Integration

Much remains untapped by the frayed connections that divide sacred from secular in our culture. But the foundation for cooperation between faith and science is strong, and when medicine and the church work together for good, combining the hope for salvation with the pursuit of health can have some astounding effects for the entire community.

Christian Community Development

On the west side of Chicago are Lawndale Community Church and Lawndale Christian Health Center. Lawndale Community Church decided early on in its history to care about health. So the health center was started, but only as one part of the church's larger commitment to the health and well-being of its neighbors. Over a number of years, the neighborhood had declined, neglected by the larger society around it, leaving poor schools, violent streets, few jobs, several liquor stores, one grocery store, and numerous places to buy lottery tickets. When there is little hope, winning the lottery seems to be one's best chance. So the church made its mission to restore hope in the neighborhood by caring about everything that affects health, including housing, education, jobs, safety, and, of course, health care. Let me offer two examples of what that looks like.

Too frequently and much too young, men in this community were dying violent deaths. The church held funerals for them, some only teenagers who had been shot and killed in the spray of gang violence. The church mourned these losses and the low value of life that was demonstrated, but it did not stop there. The church reached out to the youth of the community and formed a family of care that communicated to each one, in ways spoken and unspoken, that they were important. In one sense everything the church did, from rejuvenated housing to after-school education to a health center that provided quality health care for all, was for this grand purpose—to show that God loves the world and every life in it, no matter who you are. The church knew that after learning to value your own life, you will begin to value others. And very slowly, after many years, the men of the church, no longer wanting to hurt others with things like guns, began helping the community with things like college education.[14]

Then there was Sandra, who was three months pregnant when she came to the health center. She had been in an abusive relationship but had left that man and was now alone. Wanting the baby but afraid of being pregnant without support, she wondered if she should have an abortion. The health center and church were in the same building, so it was easy for the doctor to ask the pastor for help. It turned out that a nursing student in the church wanted to follow and observe a pregnant woman as part of her training.

Sandra received her prenatal care at the health center, and the student was with her for all those months. Sandra also started coming to church on Sunday, which helped her feel that she was part of a family. And on the night of delivery the nursing student was there, and so too was the doctor she had come to know and trust from the many prenatal visits at the health center. And when the moment came to welcome her child into the world, though she was still a little afraid, she was not alone.[15]

Conclusion

The Recovery of Wonder

The doctor's report was simple and straightforward. A young boy, an only child, had been suffering from recurrent attacks. According to the father, his son would suddenly scream, fall to the ground in convulsions, and foam at the mouth. Happening more frequently and getting worse, it was as if they were consuming him, making the father desperate and fearful for his son's life.

This case report by a physician of the first century, Dr. Luke, the writer of the third Gospel, is clinically precise and detailed (Luke 9:37–43). It is even comprehensive enough to include the effect of the illness on the family, something that we easily forget. From the account in their Gospels our other reporters, Matthew and Mark, mention that the convulsions were strong enough to throw the boy into the water or the fire, with the life-threatening possibility that he could drown or be severely burned. Mark also made note that the attacks brought about rigidity of the body and grinding of his teeth (Matt. 17:14–18; Mark 9:14–27).

The description of the condition, recurrent seizures in a young boy, is most assuredly epilepsy. But though the diagnosis is clear, the treatment ends up being anything but standard. In first-century Palestine, the cause was thought to be a supernatural power that was throwing this boy into convulsions. In this context, Jesus "treats" the child by casting out the spirit and healing him.[1] When the people saw the boy given back to his father seizure-free, "they were all amazed at the greatness of God" (Luke 9:43).

In our day, epilepsy has a more scientific explanation related to abnormal brain waves on an electroencephalogram. The modern treatment menu includes numerous antiseizure medicines, creating a seizure-free life for many who have epilepsy. So why are most of my patients who are freed of seizures by medication so "unamazed," while people in Jesus's time were so ready to acknowledge the marvelous goodness of God?

The Loss of Wonder

To be sure, Jesus's healing of seizures was far more dramatic than our treatment of epilepsy. It happened in a moment, no daily medication was required, and prior to this most people had no recourse but to live with and suffer from the problem. But then if today's patients knew that not everyone lives seizure-free on medicines, and many continue to suffer from intractable seizures despite trying everything, they would likely be more thankful.

But a bigger problem lies beneath our current attitude toward good things. Because we have learned to take things for granted, we have ceased to marvel. This loss of wonder, as novelist and literary critic Edmund Fuller writes, is itself a sickness that weakens the human spirit:

> When awe and wonder depart from our awareness, depression sets in, and after its blanket has lain smotheringly upon us for a while, despair may ensue, or the quest for kicks begin. The loss of wonder, of awe, of the sense of the sublime, is a condition leading to the death of the soul. There is no more withering state than that which takes all things for granted, whether with respect to human beings or to the rest of the natural order.[2]

Taking health and medicine for granted, withering our sense of wonder, derives from the colossal success of modern science and its associated technology. In effusive moments we speak of the "miracles" of medicine, but our underlying assumption is that these miracles are founded on scientific understandings that are under our control. The sciences by their nature cease to wonder to the extent to which they attain results. The better our results, the less we wonder or marvel at their success.

One of the strongest effects of this commitment to a mechanical assessment of reality is a split between nature and supernature. This split "generates the modern concept of the 'miracle'; a kind of punctual hole blown in the regular order of things from outside."[3] The regular order, bound within the immanent frame, being fully knowable, is neither miraculous nor mysterious. The supernatural is left outside, to break in upon the regular order of disenchanted nature on rare occasions. But limiting the supernatural to an intervention or violation of the natural world hinders our proper sense of awe and wonder, as ethicist Allen Verhey explains:

> We are on a dangerous path if we allow this contrast of the "natural" and the "supernatural" to empty the world of wonder, if we use it to define a miracle simply as a contradiction of nature, or if we understand "nature" itself as *without God* and the power of God. Science may indeed say many true and important things about nature without using God as a hypothesis, but all that it says should nurture a sense of awe, not just a sense of mastery.[4]

To have a sense of awe, to see the extraordinary in the ordinary, means that it is "precisely the ordinary operation of things which constitutes the 'miracle.'"[5] But in order to understand what usually happens as a miracle, we would need to accept that what *usually* happens does not *always* happen. And for that we would need a different attitude, to be sure a more humble one, about how much we think we know.

To Know in Part

A "take it for granted" attitude is based on a belief that what we know is complete, and when we act on this complete understanding, we can be certain that what we expect to happen will happen. Though we know now more than we knew before, specifically in the realm of science, knowing more is never the same as knowing all. And no matter how much we know, it will always be in part, and if truth be told, always a much smaller part than we realize.

Since we never fully know, the good outcome is never an always nor the bad outcome ever a never. But facing the truth that we know in part allows a healthy sense of wonder to return, for it is only the one who does not fully know who "wonders," as philosopher Josef Pieper points out:

> To wonder is not to know fully, not to conceive absolutely; it means not to know what is behind it all; it means, as Aquinas says, "that the cause of that at which we wonder is hidden from us." And so, to wonder is not to know, not to know fully, not to be able to conceive. To conceive a thing, to possess comprehensive and exhaustive knowledge of a thing, is to cease to wonder.[6]

Being freed from the illusion of knowing fully opens us up to other and richer possibilities:

> The sense of wonder certainly deprives the mind of those penultimate certainties that we had up till now taken for granted. . . . But further than that, wonder signifies that the world is profounder, more all-embracing and mysterious than the logic of everyday reason had taught us to believe. The innermost feeling of wonder is fulfilled in a deepened sense of mystery.[7]

In lieu of thinking we possess complete knowledge, our wonder becomes a longing for knowledge, the searching for truth,[8] but with an inward awareness that one does not fully know and cannot fully control. Rather, we are *viatores*, beings on the way, in search of truth, but who are "not yet."[9] The end result of this receptive attitude to reality is joy:

> Perhaps one might risk the following proposition. Wherever there is spiritual joy, wonder will also be found; and wherever the capacity for joy exists the capacity for wonder will be found. The joy that accompanies wonder is the joy of the beginner, of the mind and spirit that is always open to what is fresh, new, and as yet unknown.[10]

With a mixture of wonder and joy, the people marveled at the healing of the boy with epilepsy. With that same mixture, we too can marvel when our medicines work or our tissues heal after an operation. Knowing in part, we are grateful for the control of health we have, though it is only in part. Sometimes, for reasons no one understands, though we should have gotten better, we don't. At other times, we get better for no reason from an illness that no one quite understood. Besides the capacity to marvel when things go well, our openness to surprise allows the distinct and important possibility of joy and wonder even in the midst of unanticipated and/or undesired outcomes, where in weakness and suffering we still have hope from unexpected places or in unexpected ways.

How else to comprehend a woman addicted to amphetamines, failing all prior efforts and programs to get clean, who becomes pregnant and for the sake of her baby suddenly stops using drugs? Or a young mother in Africa who dies of tuberculosis but dies grateful that her little baby will be adopted by an infertile couple who gets to know joy they thought they would never have? Or a man who, realizing he only has a few months to live after the diagnosis of cancer, finally reaches out to ask forgiveness and repair the broken family relationships he long ago severed by his youthful behavior and dies in peace surrounded by loved ones? Accepting that we know only in part, we remain open to surprise, and the very fact of our anticipation keeps us alert to awe we might otherwise miss.

The apostle Paul, writing to the church at Corinth, understood that whatever we know now, it will always be in part: "For now we see only a reflection as in a mirror; then we shall see face to face. Now I know in part; then I shall know fully, even as I am fully known" (1 Cor. 13:12). Knowing in part, we strive for truth and remain open to wonder and surprise, believing that one day we will know fully— and more wonderful than that, also be fully known. In the meantime the best we can hope is to know in part and be known in part. But even that is a risky venture.

Why Should Humpty Come Down?

After all our exploring, we return to Humpty, who turned down Alice's invitation to come down from his wall.

> "Why do you sit out here all alone?" said Alice, not wishing to begin an argument.

"Why, because there's nobody with me!" cried Humpty Dumpty. "Did you think I didn't know the answer to *that*? Ask another."

"Don't you think you'd be safer down on the ground?" Alice went on, not with any idea of making another riddle, but simply in her good-natured anxiety for the queer creature. "That wall is so *very* narrow!"[11]

Though the wall was "so very narrow," Humpty felt safer where he was, alone but assuming all would be well, and trusting in the king's rescue if anything happened.

But whether Humpty accepts it or not, life is more uncertain than he imagines and remains full of mystery and surprise. If we were to coax him down, it wouldn't be because life on the ground is necessarily safer or more certain. It couldn't be because he would feel less vulnerable or in control. It wouldn't be because he would know more, possess more, live longer, or live better. But if Humpty did come down, he would no longer be alone. Life alone is always more risky than life with others. Life alone is always more fearful, more closed to wonder, and more restricted in joy. And life alone will always fail, because only in community can full healing and health happen, as our final story shows.

Table Fellowship

It occurs every Thursday night at Christ House in Washington, DC, a residential facility for sick, homeless men and women who need ongoing medical and nursing care in a safe place where they can recuperate. Some stay a few days, some a few months, and some enter long-term programs over many years. But on Thursday night, it is a simple, shared meal around tables, residents and staff and church members who eat and worship together.

First, there is a large meal, more than enough for everyone, prepared by a visiting group in the adjacent kitchen and served family style. As the dessert is served, one of the residents sits down at the piano. Only recently arrived, he is partially blind but able to tap out gospel music with so much joy that everyone starts clapping and singing. As the plates are cleared, the pastor begins a short service. He offers another form of nourishment around another table, the Table of the Lord, surrounding it with words of liturgy and an atmosphere of reverence that draws everyone together in a quiet moment. After the bread and juice are shared, all that is left is one more song. But not before Harvey stands up and has his say.

Harvey has already been at Christ House for many months. When he was young, his father hit him in the head with a monkey wrench, causing permanent brain damage and recurrent seizures. He went to a lot of church when he was little, but no one knew if he was getting anything out of it. Treated as if he were dumb, he didn't finish school, left home, and ended up homeless in Washington, DC, drinking many nights and sleeping in the cold. Occasionally the health van would come by to see if Harvey needed anything. But Harvey wanted nothing from anyone. He no longer wanted to take the risk of trusting anyone. It was safer to be alone and isolated, because everything he had experienced told him he was nothing and no one cared. And one night, as if to confirm what he believed, some kids came to where he was lying, doused him with gasoline, and set him on fire.

Harvey was unconscious when they took him to the hospital, where he needed skin grafts and weeks of intensive care. But finally he was ready for discharge and came to Christ House. As the wounds of his body healed, the unconditional care and underlying affirmation of his human dignity embedded in the daily routines of the staff touched deeper wounds. Harvey slowly came down off his wall and began to let people see his true self. After his medical needs were resolved, he stayed and joined the programs that would eventually get him off the street and into his own apartment. Harvey especially liked the church activities and came to all its gatherings. It turned out he had gotten a lot more out of church when he was young than anyone realized.

And now he stands up this Thursday night, with his toothless smile and that crazy look in his eyes. Anywhere else, people would have thought he was crazy. But the church had learned that Harvey had unique spiritual insight. And Harvey learned that this was one place where people listen to him. Once again, as had happened before, his simple but stirring words come as if from the mouth of God, telling each one of God's love. And all the people say, "Amen!" Then they sing a song and file out, filled with wonder at all they have seen and heard as they head back to work, back to home, or back to bed.

Notes

Preface

1. Edmund Fuller, "A Critic's Notes," *Wall Street Journal*, May 5, 1987, 34.

Introduction

1. Average life expectancy was less than forty years at the time of Virgil. It is important to note that life expectancy in these early years was heavily influenced by infant mortality, which could exceed 30 percent. Health risks continued high for most of childhood; but for those who survived childhood, their life span, more particular to the individual than life expectancy, which is a population parameter, could easily be sixty years and beyond. Thus there is no disagreement between limited life expectancy and the presence of older people in the population. Life expectancy is a useful measurement because it is commonly available and therefore helpful for comparison.

2. National Health Expenditure Accounts, Centers for Medicare and Medicaid Services, 2014, accessed January 19, 2015, http://www.cms.gov/Research -Statistics-Data-and-Systems/Statistics-Trends-and-Reports/NationalHealth ExpendData/NationalHealthAccountsHistorical.html.

3. Estimates come from a variety of sources: Geoff Williams, "The Heavy Price of Losing Weight," *U.S. News and World Report*, January 2, 2013, accessed October 9, 2015, http://money.usnews.com/money/personal-finance/articles /2013/01/02/the-heavy-price-of-losing-weight; "Americans Spent More Than 12 Billion in 2014," *American Society for Aesthetic Plastic Surgery*, March 11, 2015, accessed October 9, 2015, http://www.surgery.org/media/news-releases /the-american-society-for-aesthetic-plastic-surgery-reports-americans-spent -more-than-12-billion-in-2014—pro; "10 Things the Beauty Industry Won't Tell You," *Market Watch,* April 20, 2011, accessed October 9, 2015, http:// www.marketwatch.com/story/10-things-the-beauty-industry-wont-tell-you -1303249279432.

4. Donald M. Berwick and Andrew D. Hackbarth, "Eliminating Waste in US Health Care," *Journal of the American Medical Association* 307 (2012): 1,513–16.

5. The enactment of the Affordable Care Act in 2010 has altered this trend, but it does not change the general phenomenon.

6. Institute of Medicine, *America's Uninsured Crisis: Consequences for Health and Health Care* (Washington, DC: National Academies Press, 2009), 60–63.

7. Organization for Economic Co-operation and Development, OECD Health Statistics 2014, accessed January 19, 2015, http://www.oecd.org/els/health-systems/health-data.htm.

8. The Democratic Republic of Congo stands as a representative of the poorest countries in the world, many of which are found in sub-Saharan Africa. This data and more is updated and available at Health Care Expenditure per Capita, *The World Bank*, accessed December 26, 2014, http://data.worldbank.org/indicator/SH.XPD.PCAP.

9. One study that tracked the use of time by emergency-room physicians throughout a day's work found they spent 43 percent of their time on data entry and 28 percent of their time with patients, with most of the rest spent reviewing test results and conversing with colleagues. Total mouse clicks approached four thousand in a busy ten-hour day. See Robert G. Hill, Lynn Marie Sears, and Scott W. Melanson, "4000 Clicks: A Productivity Analysis of Electronic Medical Records in a Community Hospital ED," *American Journal of Emergency Medicine* 31 (2013): 1,591–94.

10. Sir John Denham (1615–1669), "The Progress of Learning," in *Poems and Translations in with Sophy*, accessed October 20, 2015, http://quod.lib.umich.edu/cgi/t/text/text-idx?c=eebo;idno=A35654.

Chapter 1: Taking Control of Health

1. Lewis Carroll, *Alice's Adventures in Wonderland and Through the Looking-Glass* (New York: Schocken, 1979), 171.

2. Ibid., 176.

3. Charles Taylor, *A Secular Age* (Cambridge, MA: Belknap Press, 2007), 542.

4. Though Taylor's focus is the modern West, he clearly believes that the secularity he describes, though originating in the West, is extending beyond to influence our entire global context. Consider China and Russia as two large examples.

5. Taylor, *Secular Age*, 15.

6. Many would argue that background assumptions are especially dangerous for those who refuse to acknowledge their influence.

7. Taylor spends considerable time describing a range of "cross pressures" that can challenge the framework and question the sufficiency of the immanent frame as an explanation for life. For that reason, most people do not live every day as if the frame is completely closed. Holes in the frame, an "open take," allow many to find meaning in life from sources that a purely "closed" frame does not permit, including God, the spirits, magical forces, etc. Interestingly, there are certain contexts where a closed frame is so dominant that it overwhelms the individual's usual preferences. Technologically oriented biomedicine represents one of those contexts, as we will see.

8. Stephen Pastis, "Pearls Before Swine," *Denver Post*, July 19, 2009.

9. Ibid.

10. Taylor, *Secular Age*, 37–38.

11. Ibid., 35.

12. The predictability of the universe is the ground upon which our modern scientific enterprise is built. Though it is somewhat artificial to separate it from the view of self that is discussed in this chapter, because it is central to our topic

of health and medicine, we will reserve the entire next chapter to it. Suffice it to say that the Enlightenment Scientific Project was nowhere near satisfied with understanding how the universe operated—this knowledge must be used to gain power over it.

13. Taylor, *Secular Age*, 539.
14. Ibid., 300.
15. Ibid., 580–89.
16. Ibid., 38.
17. Quoted in ibid., 588.
18. In modern ethics, we are restricted only by the "harm principle": no one has a right to interfere with me for my own good, except to prevent harm to others. Otherwise, if I consent or authorize it, it can be done.
19. Taylor, *Secular Age*, 299.
20. Ibid., 490.
21. The first report of an association between a prenatal maternal blood test, serum alpha-fetoprotein, and a fetal abnormality, trisomy 18, appeared in 1984, setting the stage for the multiplicity of prenatal testing options that have followed. See I. R. Merkatz et al., "An Association between Low Maternal Serum Alpha-Fetoprotein and Fetal Chromosomal Abnormalities," *American Journal of Obstetrics and Gynecology* 148 (1984): 886–94.
22. Chromosomal microarray analysis (CMA) has the ability to scan the genes of a fetus at one hundred times the detail of current testing, revealing far more potential health risks than current prenatal testing.
23. An early study on the use of this technology reveals that women reported so much anxiety about the health of their fetus for the duration of the pregnancy that the results were experienced as unwanted "toxic" knowledge. See B. A. Bernhardt et al., "Women's Experiences Receiving Abnormal Prenatal Chromosomal Microarray Testing Results," *Genetics in Medicine* 15 (2013): 139–45.

Chapter 2: The Desire for Certainty in an Uncertain World

1. Especially concerning in light of these past events is recent news of outbreaks of measles in several communities, highlighting the serious consequences of vaccine refusal on the part of many families. Reducing "herd immunity," it endangers the extreme reduction in vaccine-preventable disease that has been accomplished in the last decades in the United States. What seems odd to some is the decision of an increasing number of families to forgo the benefit of this scientific achievement. The best way to understand this behavior is to realize what people currently fear. Never having seen the dangers of these diseases, they fear something much less likely—the rare side effects of the vaccine. We will look later at the manipulation of our fears stemming from our dependence on any study that appears "scientific."
2. Michael Bliss, *William Osler: A Life in Medicine* (New York: Oxford University Press, 1999), 155.
3. Ibid., 283.
4. Romano Guardini, *The End of the Modern World* (Wilmington, DE: ISI Books, 1998), 24.
5. Harvey published his findings in 1628 in a monograph entitled *De Motu*

Cordis. Through direct observation and experimentation of animal anatomy and physiology, Harvey determined the way blood coursed through the body and forever changed the view of modern science.

6. Steven Shapin, *The Scientific Revolution* (Chicago: University of Chicago Press, 1996), 68–69.

7. Ibid., 60.

8. Ibid., 150; emphasis original.

9. Charles Taylor, *A Secular Age* (Cambridge, MA: Belknap Press, 2007), 40, 270–95.

10. Mention must be made of Francis Bacon, one of the fathers of the modern scientific method. He was one of the first and firmest believers in the use of scientific method for the sake of human welfare. Among his famous quotes: "Knowledge is power" and should be used for the "relief of Man's estate." For further discussion of the influence of Baconian Project on modern medicine, see Allen Verhey, *Reading the Bible in the Strange World of Medicine* (Grand Rapids, MI: Eerdmans, 2003).

11. Bliss, *William Osler*, 393.

12. "Man's Redemption of Man: A Lay Sermon by William Osler," accessed March 6, 2015. The full address may be found at http://www.gutenberg.org/files/36926/36926-h/36926-h.htm.

13. Ibid.; emphasis original.

14. Ibid.

15. Quote attributed to Paul Ramsey, cited in Courtney S. Campbell, "Religion and Moral Meaning in Bioethics," *Hastings Center Report* 20 (July/August 1990): 6.

16. Laurie Becklund, "As I Lay Dying," February 20, 2015, accessed March 12, 2015, http://www.latimes.com/opinion/op-ed/la-oe-becklund-breast-cancer-komen-20150222-story.html#page=1.

17. To experience the patient's sense of failure as our own can be dangerous ground for any doctor, nurse, or member of the health care team. For many, it causes us to run. Patient abandonment by health caregivers when cure is no longer possible is a common problem. Though this has prompted new efforts to improve medical training in chronic care and palliative care, the temptation to flee in the face of perceived failure remains high. For some, they simply give up. Though there are a range of factors, failing to meet patients' expectations—and hidden within that is our own false expectations that we can deliver what patients want—is contributing to the loss of many from the practice of medicine at alarming rates. See the Physicians Foundation, "A Survey of American Physicians: Practice Patterns and Perspectives," September 2012, accessed October 9, 2015, http://www.physiciansfoundation.org/uploads/default/Physicians_Foundation_2012_Biennial_Survey.pdf).

18. Erwin Chargaff, *Heraclitean Fire: Sketches From a Life Before Nature* (New York: Rockefeller University Press, 1978), 120.

19. Ibid.

20. Ibid.

21. Ibid., 106.

22. Ibid., 123.

23. Ibid., 172.
24. Dorothy Sayers, *The Mind of the Maker* (San Francisco: HarperCollins, 1987), 194.
25. Ibid., 188.
26. Ibid., 195.
27. There remain many pockets in the world, like sub-Saharan Africa, where early childhood mortality continues to be high, mimicking rates experienced in the United States over seventy-five years ago. But for most economically developed nations, with advances in the safety of birth and early childhood, most of us count on a healthy delivery and safe passage during the first year of life. See *Levels and Trends in Child Mortality*, report by the United Nations Children's Fund, 2012.
28. S. M. Taffel, P. J. Placek, T. Liss, "Trends in the United States Cesarean Section Rate and Reasons for the 1980–85 Rise," *American Journal of Public Health* 77 (1987): 955–59.
29. J. A. Martin et al., "Births: Final Data for 2009," National Vital Statistics Reports, 60 no. 1 (Hyattsville, MD: National Center for Health Statistics, 2011).
30. Emma L. Barber et al., "Contributing Indications to the Rising Cesarean Delivery Rate," *Obstetrics and Gynecology* 118 (2011): 29–38.
31. Jonathan Swift, *Gulliver's Travels* (Roslyn, NY: Walter J. Black, 1932), 169–70.
32. Psychological research on decision making under the shadow of risk and uncertainty has shown that we weight small probabilities based on our affective state of hope or fear. Fear and dread make small probabilities of risk loom large, while being positively inclined to anticipate a good outcome leads us to overestimate benefit. This divergence between our emotional reactions to a risky situation and more objective cognitive evaluations of risk severity and probability explain many of our responses when faced with decisions about health and disease. When we take lifelong medicine when healthy to reduce the risk of a bad outcome, our hope inclines us to overestimate benefit. On the other hand, when we get an abnormal result of a screening exam for cancer, though the likelihood of cancer remains very low, we are very anxious while we await a biopsy for conclusive results. Our fear of this dreaded outcome makes us very sensitive to the possibility and much less influenced by the unlikely probability. See G. F. Loewenstein et al., "Risk as Feelings," *Psychological Bulletin* 127 (2001): 267–86.
33. S. F. Katz and M. Morrow, "Contralateral Prophylactic Mastectomy for Breast Cancer: Addressing Peace of Mind," *Journal of the American Medical Association* 310 (2013): 793–94. Since there is nearly universal coverage for this procedure regardless of level of cancer risk and benefit, most surgeons find it difficult to refuse a patient's request, even if they believe it is of no value. If failure to accede to patients' desires is made public, such as through social media, the doctor may lose future patients. This twist in the cord of doctor-patient relationship that overemphasizes patient autonomy in the name of patient-centered care is good neither for the patient nor for the health care system.

34. Luc Ferry, *A Brief History of Thought: A Philosophical Guide to Living* (New York: HarperCollins, 2011), 212.

35. Ibid., 215–16.

36. Peter Augustine Lawler, *Stuck with Virtue: The American Individual and Our Biotechnological Future* (Wilmington, DE: ISI Books, 2005), 168.

37. Taylor, *Secular Age*, 143.

38. Quoted in David Bosch, *Transforming Mission: Paradigm Shifts in the Theology of Mission* (Maryknoll, NY: Orbis, 1991), 274.

39. Wendell Berry, *The Way of Ignorance* (Washington, DC: Shoemaker & Hoard, 2005), 77.

Chapter 3: As It Was in the Beginning

1. Erik H. Erikson and Joan M. Erikson, *The Life Cycle Completed* (New York: Norton, 1997), 56–57.

2. Glenn Tinder, *The Fabric of Hope* (Grand Rapids, MI: Eerdmans, 2001), 140.

3. The word *humble*, derived from the Latin root *humus*, i.e., "of the earth," and related to humus, the dark, organic material of soil, further connects this sober view of ourselves to the earthly origin of our nature.

4. Quoted in David Cayley, *The Rivers North of the Future: The Testament of Ivan Illich* (Toronto: House of Anansi, 2005), 74.

5. Augustine, *Concerning the City of God against the Pagans*, trans. Henry Bettenson (London: Penguin, 2003), bk. 20, chap. 20 (p. 937).

6. Gilbert Meilaender, *The Freedom of a Christian* (Grand Rapids, MI: Brazos Press, 2006), 119–35.

7. Dietrich Bonhoeffer, *Creation and Fall: A Theological Interpretation of Genesis 1–3*, trans. John C. Fletcher (New York: MacMillan, 1959), 44.

8. J. L. Natoli et al., "Prenatal Diagnosis of Down Syndrome: A Systematic Review of Termination Rates (1995–2011)," *Prenatal Diagnosis* 32 (2012): 142–53.

9. M. J. Korenromp et al., "Maternal Decision to Terminate Pregnancy in Case of Down Syndrome," *American Journal of Obstetrics and Gynecology* 196 (2007): 149.e1–11.

10. B. G. Skotko, S. P. Levine, R. Goldstein, "Having a Son or Daughter with Down Syndrome: Perspectives from Mothers and Fathers," *American Journal of Medical Genetics* 155 (2011): 2,335–47; B. G. Skotko, S. P. Levine, R. Goldstein, "Having a Brother or Sister with Down Syndrome: Perspectives from Siblings," *American Journal of Medical Genetics* 155 (2011): 2,348–59. B. G. Skotko, S. P. Levine, R. Goldstein, "Self-perceptions from People with Down Syndrome," *American Journal of Medical Genetics* 155 (2011): 2,360–69. These three studies were conducted by Boston Children's Hospital. In the first study, out of 2,044 parents or guardians surveyed, 79 percent reported their outlook on life was "more positive" because of their child with Down syndrome. A second study found that among siblings of children with Down syndrome, 97 percent expressed feelings of pride for their brother or sister, and 88 percent were convinced that they were better people because of their sibling. This study polled siblings over the age of twelve. A third study focused on the feelings and attitudes of people with Down syndrome. Among adults with Down syndrome, 99 percent said they were happy with their lives, and

97 percent said they liked who they were. Ninety-six percent said they liked the way they looked.

11. For some, the measure of success for the prenatal diagnosis of Down syndrome would be a future world in which no baby would be born with this "imperfection." Such matters of life and death affect us all. If Jean Vanier's life in community with those with mental and physical disabilities can give any guidance, "it is people who are weak, rejected, marginalized, counted as useless, who can become a source of life and of salvation for us as individuals as well as for our world." Jean Vanier, *From Brokenness to Community* (Mahwah, NJ: Paulist Press, 1992), 10. Or, to put it another way, "The eye cannot say to the hand, 'I don't need you!' And the head cannot say to the feet, 'I don't need you!' On the contrary, those parts of the body that seem to be weaker are indispensable" (1 Cor. 12:21–22). All of us in a caring society should be deeply concerned about losing parts of the body indispensable for being fully human.

12. Bonhoeffer, *Creation and Fall*, 49.

13. Ibid., 51.

14. Ibid., 53.

15. Romano Guardini, *The End of the Modern World* (Wilmington, DE: ISI Books, 1998), 33.

16. Pre-traumatic stress disorder, in contrast to post-traumatic stress disorder (PTSD) that comes after a traumatic event, has been bandied around as a term to describe the mental anguish that results from preparing for the worst before it actually happens. This form of PTSD can affect many more people, since it can exist and persist though the event never happens.

17. C. S. Lewis, *The World's Last Night and Other Essays* (New York: Harcourt Brace Jovanovich, 1960), 105–6.

Chapter 4: Disembodiment in Health Care, Part 1

1. F. Peabody, "The Care of the Patient," *Journal of the American Medical Association* 88 (1927): 877. The full article is available on-line: http://courses.washington.edu/hmed665i/MSJAMA_Landmark_Article_The_Care_of_the_Patient.html.

2. Ibid., 878.

3. C. S. Lewis, *The Abolition of Man* (New York: HarperCollins, 2001), 69.

4. Charles Taylor, *A Secular Age* (Cambridge, MA: Belknap Press, 2007), 285, 595.

5. Ibid., 746.

6. Ibid.

7. This story is from Sherwin B. Nuland, *Doctors: The Biography of Medicine* (New York: Vintage, 1988), 219–28.

8. Quoted in ibid., 220.

9. Quoted in ibid.

10. The term *gnosticism* is derived from *gnosis*, meaning "knowledge." A core understanding of gnosticism is that salvation comes through knowledge.

11. Philip J. Lee, *Against the Protestant Gnostics* (New York: Oxford University Press, 1987), 8.

12. Ibid., 7.

13. Wendell Berry, *What Are People For?* (San Francisco: North Point Press, 1990), 190–91.

14. Stephanie Saul, "Building a Baby, with Few Ground Rules," *New York Times*, December 13, 2009, accessed September 19, 2015, http://www.nytimes.com /2009/12/13/us/13surrogacy.html?_r=0.

15. In 2009 a report issued by the Mayday Fund entitled "A Call to Revolutionize Chronic Pain in America: An Opportunity in Health Care Reform" was endorsed by more than forty professional medical organizations. It appropriately recognized the large number of people suffering from chronic pain in the United States—up to 25 percent of the population according to their studies—but at the same time made pain a treatable disease. Accessed April 28, 2015, http://maydaypainreport.org/report.php.

16. R. K. Portenoy and K. M. Foley, "Chronic Use of Opioid Analgesics in Nonmalignant Pain: Report of 38 Cases," *Pain* 25 (1986): 171–86.

17. "Injury Prevention and Control: Prescription Drug Overdose," *Centers for Disease Control and Prevention*, March 16, 2016, accessed April 9, 2016, http://www.cdc.gov/drugoverdose/data/prescribing.html.

18. Nicholas B. King et al., "Determinants of Increased Opioid-Related Mortality in the United States and Canada, 1990–2013: A Systematic Review," *American Journal of Public Health* 104 (2014): e32–e42.

19. From 2000–2010, 75 percent of persons newly initiating heroin reported having started the abuse of opiates with a prescription drug. This is a near complete reversal from a comparison group in the 1960s, when over 80 percent used heroin as the initial opiate of abuse. See T. J. Cicero et al., "The Changing Face of Heroin Use in the United States: A Retrospective Analysis of the Past 50 Years," *Journal of the American Medical Association Psychiatry* 71 (2014): 821–26.

20. Center for Disease Control and Prevention, "Increases in Drug and Opioid Overdose Deaths—United States, 2000–2014," *Morbidity and Mortality Weekly Report* 64 (2016): 1,378–82.

21. G. M. Franklin, "Opioids for Chronic Noncancer Pain: A Position Paper of the American Academy of Neurology," *Neurology* 83 (2014): 1,277–84.

22. Jeffrey Bishop, *The Anticipatory Corpse* (Notre Dame, IN: University of Notre Dame Press, 2011), 49–60.

23. George L. Engel, "The Need for a New Medical Model: A Challenge for Biomedicine," *Science* 196 (1977): 132.

24. Bishop, *Anticipatory Corpse*, 235–52.

25. I am referring to ICD coding, which is for the purpose of billing based on diagnostic categories. If coding is not done correctly, the medical system will not be paid.

Chapter 5: Disembodiment in Health Care, Part 2

1. From the report of a committee of four mathematicians to the Academy of Sciences in Paris in 1835 on a statistical comparison of the success of two different operations for the removal of gallstones. Quote taken from Ian Hacking, *The Taming of Chance* (New York: Cambridge University Press, 1990), 81.

2. Gary Taubes and Charles C. Mann, "Epidemiology Faces Its Limits," *Science* 269 (1995): 167.

3. ELF-EMF is extremely low-frequency electric and magnetic fields.

4. Gary Zeman, "Health Risks Associated with Living Near High Voltage Power

Lines," *Health Physics Society*, August 13, 2014, accessed September 16, 2015, http://hps.org/hpspublications/articles/powerlines.html.

5. "Heavy Cell Phone Use Can Quadruple Your Risk of Brain Cancer," accessed September 16, 2015, http://articles.mercola.com/sites/articles/archive/2015/01/06/cell-phone-use-brain-cancer-risk.aspx.

6. Quoted in Hacking, *Taming of Chance*, 82.

7. Quoted in ibid., 83.

8. Ibid., 84.

9. Ibid., 1.

10. Jeffrey Bishop, *The Anticipatory Corpse* (Notre Dame, IN: University of Notre Dame Press, 2011), 79.

11. Dostoyevsky, the champion of the individual conscience, gives a warning for all ages of the dangers of a science of human beings that eliminates their humanity. As he wrote: "But there is one very puzzling thing: how does it come about that all the statisticians and experts and lovers of humanity, when they enumerate the good things of life, always omit one particular one? One's own free and unfettered volition . . . is never taken into consideration because it will not fit any classification, and the omission of which always sends all systems and theories to the devil." Quoted in Hacking, *Taming of Chance*, 146.

12. Hippocrates, *The Theory and Practice of Medicine* (New York: Citadel Press, 1964), 42.

13. Ibid., 44.

14. Stephen J. Gould, "The Median Isn't the Message," *Discover* 6 (1985): 40–42.

15. Gould, "The Median," 41.

16. Paul Kalanithi, *When Breath Becomes Air* (New York: Random House, 2016), 134–35.

17. Hacking, *Taming of Chance*, 169.

18. Allan V. Horwitz and Jerome C. Wakefield, *The Loss of Sadness: How Psychiatry Transformed Normal Sorrow into Depressive Disorder* (New York: Oxford University Press, 2007).

19. Comparing the period 1988–1994 with the period 2004–2008, the use of antidepressants increased fivefold in people over eighteen in the United States. During the period 2005–2008, antidepressants became the third most common prescription drug taken by Americans of all ages. See "Health, United States, 2010: With Special Feature on Death and Dying" (Hyattsville, MD: National Center for Health Statistics, 2011), 19.

20. "Anti-Depressant Use in Persons Age 12 and Over: United States, 2005–2008," NCHS Data Brief, No. 76, October 2011, accessed May 8, 2015, http://www.cdc.gov/nchs/data/databriefs/db76.htm. One wonders how far we will go, and if in the process we will lose the creativity formed from wrestling with the depth of human emotions, seen in authors such as Ernest Hemingway and Leo Tolstoy, or painters such as Vincent van Gogh, or spiritual mentors such as St. Theresa of Avila and Henri Nouwen. Would the world be a poorer place for having pursued this agenda with such vigor? It brings to mind Aldous Huxley's dystopic novel *A Brave New World*. Whenever people began to struggle with their thoughts or wonder if there were something more, the Controllers would give them a dose of Soma. One swallow and the negative

feelings were dispelled, only to awake the next morning with everything back to normal, permitting society to continue just as it was and always will be. This is a chilling thought, but one that grows more possible when people's emotional experiences are reduced to dots on a distribution curve and someone has the power to name what the normal at the center looks like.

21. In 2011, over 10 percent of children between the ages of four and seventeen had been diagnosed with ADHD, representing a 42 percent increase from 2003. The prevalence was even higher in high school boys, where nearly 20 percent had received an ADHD diagnosis. See: Susanna N. Visser et al., "Trends in the Parent-Report of Health Care Provider-Diagnosed and Medicated Attention-Deficit/Hyperactivity Disorder: United States, 2003–2011," *Journal of the American Academy of Child and Adolescent Psychiatry* 53 (2014): 34–46.e2. Not surprisingly, sales of stimulant medications used to treat ADHD have more than doubled, from $4 billion in 2007 to $9 billion in 2012. Besides cost, the increased number of prescriptions written for these controlled substances produces increased risk for diversion and abuse. See Alan Schwarz and Sarah Cohen, "A.D.H.D. Seen in 11% of U.S. Children as Diagnoses Rise," *New York Times*, March 31, 2013, accessed May 22, 2015, http://www.nytimes.com/2013/04/01/health/more-diagnoses-of-hyperactivity -causing-concern.html?_r=0.

22. Adele E. Clarke et al. "Biomedicalization: Technoscientific Transformations of Health, Illness, and U.S. Biomedicine," *American Sociological Review* 68 (2003): 181–82.

23. For a more comprehensive treatment of medicalization and its adaptability to changing attitudes in culture and society, see *Biohealth: Beyond Medicalization, Imposing Health* (Eugene, OR: Pickwick, 2011). Raymond Downing has done an admirable job of showing how health, increasingly understood in a commodity culture as something we work for as an individual goal, also becomes a social and moral responsibility that remains defined mostly by external standards to which all must adhere.

24. The devilish nature of this distraction is well described in *The Screwtape Letters*, C. S. Lewis's clever interpretation of a senior devil's instruction to a junior devil to keep his charge from going over to "the Enemy," who is God. Getting people to focus on the future is one of the more important methods for a junior tempter to learn. "It is far better to make them live in the Future. . . . It is unknown to them, so that in making them think about it we make them think about unrealities. . . . [The Enemy] does not want men to give their Future their hearts, to place their treasure in it. We do. . . . We want a man hagridden by the Future—haunted by visions of an imminent heaven or hell on earth—ready to break the Enemy's commands in the Present if by so doing we make him think he can attain the one or avert the other." C. S. Lewis, *The Complete C. S. Lewis Signature Classics* (New York: HarperCollins, 2002), 228.

25. The PSA (Prostate Specific Antigen) test is a blood test to screen for prostate cancer.

26. The majority of this patient vignette has been previously published. See Robert Cutillo, "Futures Management in the Exam Room: An Improbable Agenda," *Hastings Center Report* 44 (2014): 23.

27. The numbers constantly change, depending on who is doing the study and who funds it, but the broadest and least biased analyses show that it will require one thousand men to have an annual test for ten years, a total of ten thousand tests, before one man's life is saved from prostate cancer. In the meantime, many more men will have serious side effects of the treatment, including urinary incontinence and erectile dysfunction. See Roger Chou and Michael L. LeFevre, "Prostate Cancer Screening: The Evidence, the Recommendations, and the Clinical Implications," *Journal of the American Medical Association* 306 (2011): 2,721–22.

28. Joann G. Elmore and Barnett S. Kramer, "Breast Cancer Screening: Toward Informed Decisions," *Journal of the American Medical Association* 311 (2014): 1,298–99.

29. The tool can be found at http://statindecisionaid.mayoclinic.org/index.php /statin/index.

30. Charles Taylor, *The Secular Age* (Cambridge, MA: Belknap Press, 2007), 363.

31. Walter Percy, *Signposts in a Strange Land* (New York: Farrar, Straus & Giroux, 1991), 151.

32. Jonathan Swift, *Gulliver's Travels* (Roslyn, NY: Walter J. Black, 1932), 163–69.

Chapter 6: The Gaze of the Gospel

1. Charles Taylor, *A Secular Age* (Cambridge, MA: Belknap Press, 2007), 610.

2. *Gospel* comes from the Latin *evangelium* and the Greek *euangelion;* the evangelist, then, is a bearer of good news.

3. C. S. Lewis, *God in the Dock: Essays on Theology and Ethics* (Grand Rapids, MI: Eerdmans, 1970), 80.

4. See portions of Luke 1.

5. See portions of Matthew 2.

6. Henry Chadwick, *The Early Church* (New York: Penguin, 1993), 286.

7. Irenaeus, *Against Heresies*, in *The Ante-Nicene Fathers*, vol. 1, ed. Alexander Roberts and James Donaldson (Peabody, MA: Hendrickson, 1994), 3.11.3.

8. Hans Urs von Balthasar describes how well Irenaeus understood the pervasive danger of Gnosticism: "From this general description, we can see that Gnosticism is radically anti-Christian. Irenaeus, with great perspicacity, understood this, and showed it up for what it was. For him, Christianity was about the divine and spiritual Word becoming flesh and body. The redemption depends on the real Incarnation, the real suffering on the cross, and the real resurrection of the flesh. All of these are a scandal for Gnosticism." Hans Urs von Balthasar, *The Scandal of the Incarnation: Irenaeus against the Heresies* (San Francisco: Ignatius Press, 1990), 3.

9. Robertson Davies, *The Rebel Angels* (New York: Penguin, 1981), 249–50.

10. This story first appeared in Robert Cutillo, "A Life Embodied Is a Life at Risk," *The Gospel Coalition* website, May 14, 2015, accessed April 11, 2016, https://www.thegospelcoalition.org/article/life-embodied-is-life-at-risk.

11. Henry Sigerist, a physician and historian of medicine, showed how much the Christian response to sickness and suffering differed from the surrounding culture: "The position of the sick man and the physician in society was radically changed by Christianity, which came into the world as the religion of healing."

Further on he adds, "Christianity gave the sick man a position in society he never had before, a preferential position. The new religion addressed itself to the poor, the oppressed, the sinners and the sick. It addressed itself to suffering humanity and promised healing and redemption. All other ancient cults were for the clean and the pure, excluding individuals that had become impure. Christianity relieved the sick man from the burden he had carried before. He was no longer considered an inferior being." *On the History of Medicine*, ed. Felix Marti-Ibanez (New York: MD Publications, 1960), 8, 27.

12. This view always gives hope to a suffering people, that the world still has purpose and meaning, as it did in the midst of the horrors of Nazi Germany: "It remains an experience of incomparable value that we have for once learned to see the great events of world history from below, from the perspective of the excluded, the suspected, the ill-treated, the powerless, the oppressed and despised, in short, from the perspective of the suffering . . . we come to see . . . that personal suffering is a more useful key, a more fruitful principle than personal happiness for exploring the meaning of the world in contemplation and action." Dietrich Bonhoeffer, *The Bonhoeffer Reader*, ed. Clifford J. Green and Michael P. DeJonge (Minneapolis: Fortress Press, 2013), 775.

13. Dietrich Bonhoeffer, *Ethics* (Minneapolis: Fortress Press, 2009), 87.

14. Wendell Berry, *What Are People For?* (San Francisco: North Point Press, 1990), 200.

15. T. S. Eliot, *Four Quartets* (New York: Harcourt, 1943), 44.

Chapter 7: In the Shadow of Death

1. Adapted from Luke 12:16–21, substituting health for wealth. The two are connected in many ways, particularly when we pursue either of them as if our acquisition and possession of them, and protection and control over them, will give us security.

2. Blaise Pascal, *Pensées* (written c. 1660), trans. H. F. Stewart (New York: Pantheon, 1950), 83.

3. Stephen Mitchell, *Gilgamesh: A New English Version* (New York: Free Press, 2004), 71.

4. Ibid., 150–51.

5. Ibid., 159.

6. Ibid., 168.

7. Ibid., 174–75.

8. Ernest Becker, *The Denial of Death* (New York: Free Press, 1973), 69.

9. Ibid., 87.

10. See *Time* covers: September 30, 2013, "Can Google Solve Death?"; and February 21, 2011, "2045: The Year Man Becomes Immortal."

11. The cryonics movement was launched with the publication in 1962 of *The Prospect of Immortality* by Robert Ettinger. A college math and physics professor, he initially believed science would discover in his lifetime the secret of eternal youth. When he realized this was not going to happen, he turned to cryopreservation, believing that when the secrets of immortality are discovered in the future, the frozen bodies can be revived and receive all the benefits of future technology.

12. Unduly optimistic assessments of survival prospects make it difficult for pa-

tients and doctors to use the remaining time well, often focusing more on futile care to prolong life than on measures to improve the quality of remaining life. See N. A. Christakis and E. B. Lamont, "Extent and Determinants of Error in Doctors' Prognoses in Terminally Ill Patients: Prospective Cohort Study," *British Medical Journal* 320 (2000): 469–72.

13. Contrast this with a doctor's experience in a culture more aware of the reality of death: "When dealing with Africans, one must never hold out hope of recovery to the patient and his relatives if the case is really hopeless. If death occurs without warning, they conclude that the doctor did not know the disease would have this outcome because he did not diagnose it correctly. One must tell the truth to African patients without reservation. They wish to know it, and they can bear it. Death for them is something natural. They are not afraid of it, but, on the contrary, face it calmly." Albert Schweitzer, *Out of My Life and Thought*, trans. Antje Bultmann Lemke (New York: Henry Holt, 1990), 138.

14. "End of Life Constitutes Third Rail of U.S. Health Care Policy Debate," *Medicare News Group*, accessed July 31, 2015, http://www.medicarenewsgroup .com/context/understanding-medicare-blog/understanding-medicare-blog /2013/06/03/end-of-life-care-constitutes-third-rail-of-u.s.-health-care-policy -debate. See also A. S. Kelley et al., "Determinants of Medical Expenditures in the Last Six Months of Life," *Annals Internal Medicine* 154 (2011): 235–42.

15. Harlan M. Krumholz et al., "Mortality, Hospitalizations, and Expenditures for the Medicare Population Aged 65 Years or Older, 1999–2013, *Journal of the American Medical Association* 314 (2015): 355–65.

16. "Views on End-of-Life Medical Treatment," November 2013, Pew Research Council, accessed June 16, 2015, http://www.pewforum.org/2013/11/21 /views-on-end-of-life-medical-treatments/.

17. A. C. Phelps et al., "Religious Coping and the Use of Intensive Life-Prolonging Care Near Death in Patients with Advanced Cancer," *Journal of the American Medical Association* 301 (2009): 1,140–47.

18. When we believe, by the success of our technical prowess, that death is optional, there is no death by "natural causes." Attributing everything to human agency, nature "disappears through the skylight," limiting cause of death to what we do or fail to do. If we could have prevented death and do not, we have acted immorally. What we often fail to realize is that this moral obligation, rather than strengthening our connection to God, makes us prisoners of our technological choices. See Daniel Callahan, *The Troubled Dream of Life: Living with Mortality* (New York: Simon & Schuster, 1993), 57–71.

19. Leon Kass, *Life, Liberty, and the Defense of Dignity: The Challenge for Bioethics* (San Francisco: Encounter, 2002), 260–61.

20. The growth of medicine as an industry and institution is fueled by many sources. In chapter 5 we spoke of the process of medicalization. Fear of death is perhaps the most important cause; aided and abetted by public demands and medicine's confusion about its own role, hope that death can be overcome increases expectations that medicine can deliver us. But the desire to cure death can be damaging. For medical students who are familiar with the Starling curve of cardiac compensation, in the face of increased pressure the heart hypertrophies. Likewise the medical project hypertrophies under the pressure

to prevent death. The sad fact at the end of the analogy is that if the pressure remains too high for too long, the heart fails; medicine as a traditional profession of healing is failing under the pressure to defeat death.

21. Philippe Aries, *The Hour of Our Death*, trans. Helen Weaver (New York: Knopf, 1981), 592.

22. Geoffrey Gorer, *Death, Grief, and Mourning* (New York: Arno Press, 1977), 128.

23. The extension of the practice of cremation and the reduction of the social ceremony of the funeral to a more sterile and distant memorial service are further movements toward simplification and efficiency. See Aries, *Hour of Our Death*, 600.

24. Arthur C. McGill, *Death and Life: An American Theology* (Eugene, OR: Wipf & Stock, 1987), 19–20.

25. Callahan, *The Troubled Dream of Life*, 36–37.

26. Of course, the right to choose is not always defiant. When we worry about the burden we will be to others or the possibility of prolonged pain, our fear of dying becomes a fear of living, and we would prefer to end it before these things happen.

27. Charles Taylor, *A Secular Age* (Cambridge, MA: Belknap Press, 2007), 29–42.

28. See Aries, *Hour of Our Death*, 5–28.

29. Ibid., 8.

30. Ibid., 6.

31. Ibid., 7.

32. Quoted in ibid., 10.

33. Taylor, *Secular Age*, 54–56.

34. A story in Genesis reminds us of the gentle goodness of this awareness. In Genesis 49:29–33, Jacob knows the time is at hand, or as the Scriptures beautifully say, "I am about to be gathered to my people" (v. 29). With such understanding he gives instructions to help his family prepare for his departure, after which he "drew his feet up into the bed, breathed his last and was gathered to his people" (Gen. 49:33). More than just awareness, it is also understanding, acceptance, and preparation for the ways of God for human life that by nature must include death.

35. Albert Camus, *Le Mythe de Sisyphe* (Paris: Gallimard, Foloi essais, 1942), 46.

36. In Matt. 16:3–4, the religious leaders ask Jesus for a sign, something directly from heaven that will be unequivocal and clear. Jesus, marveling at their ability to predict the weather but their inability to read the signs of the times already available to them, offers them but one more sign: the sign of Jonah, referring to the three days the prophet Jonah spent in the belly of a great fish. Soon thereafter, Jesus would be three days in the grave.

Chapter 8: Death Defanged and Defeated

1. T. S. Elliot, *Murder in the Cathedral* (New York: Harcourt Brace Jovanovich, 1935).

2. Ibid., 70.

3. Ibid., 23.

4. Ibid.
5. Peter Brown, *Augustine of Hippo* (Berkeley, CA: University of California Press, 2000), 454.
6. See Matt. 16:21; 17:22; 20:17, and pars. in the other Gospels.
7. In Luke 24:13–35, two of Jesus's disciples spend several hours walking with him on the road to Emmaus and talking about all the events that had recently transpired. Yet still they are unable to recognize him until he sits and breaks bread with them at the end of the day.
8. Cyprian, "Mortality 16" (written AD 251), in *Saint Cyprian Treatises*, trans. Roy J. Deferrari (New York: Fathers of the Church, 1958), 212.
9. Rodney Stark, *The Rise of Christianity* (Princeton, NJ: Princeton University Press, 1996), 73–88.
10. Tertullian, "The Apology 39" (written AD 197), in *The Ante-Nicene Fathers*, vol. 3, ed. Alexander Roberts and James Donaldson (Peabody, MA: Hendrickson, 1994), 46.
11. C. S. Lewis, *The Weight of Glory* (New York: HarperCollins, 2001), 26.
12. It is interesting to note that the hopes of this Old Testament prophet, dating back over 2,500 years, mirror our own hopes and dreams for a new society. In fact, due to many of the advances in scientific medicine, we have already significantly reduced infant mortality and premature death. These have been good things that point to what is to come. The challenge of the resurrection is that though we continue to strive for better health and further improvements, we cannot complete the task. This should not diminish our efforts, but limit our expectations. Without recognizing those limits, we are in danger of dehumanizing the very humanity we seek to help. This comes in many forms, one of which is the unjust distribution of limited resources, which marginalizes the poor. We will take this up in the next chapter.
13. Because it is so unlike the way we would imagine it, the writers of the New Testament went out of their way to show the continued importance of the body. After Jesus rose from the dead, rather than ghostlike actions to impress his followers, the most common thing he did was eat with them. On one occasion he broke bread with them at the end of the day (Luke 24:30); another time he invited them to have breakfast in the morning (John 21:12). But the first time he meets them together illustrates it best. He is suddenly among them, and they are sure they are seeing some disembodied spirit. "Look at my hands and my feet. It is I myself! Touch me and see; a ghost does not have flesh and bones, as you see I have" (Luke 24:39). Then, in the midst of their joy and amazement, he asks the most mundane question, "'Do you have anything here to eat?' They gave him a piece of broiled fish, and he took it and ate it in their presence" (Luke 24:41–43).
14. In Phil. 3:20–21 we find the most succinct summary of this truth: "But our citizenship is in heaven. And we eagerly await a Savior from there, the Lord Jesus Christ, who, by the power that enables him to bring everything under his control, *will transform our lowly bodies so that they will be like his glorious body.*"
15. See, e.g., John 7:30; 12:32–33; and 13:1.
16. That Jesus was not a passive victim but an active participant in the drama

of his death is a distinction of utmost importance, most clearly made in John 10:17–18, "The reason my Father loves me is that I lay down my life—only to take it up again. No one takes it from me, but I lay it down of my own accord. I have authority to lay it down and authority to take it up again."

17. Dietrich Bonhoeffer, *Ethics* (Minneapolis: Fortress Press, 2009), 92.

18. Quoted in Brown, *Augustine of Hippo*, 454.

19. Philippe Aries, *Western Attitudes toward Death*, trans. Patricia M. Ranum (Baltimore: Johns Hopkins University Press, 1974), 107.

20. Daniel Callahan, *The Troubled Dream of Life: Living with Mortality* (New York: Simon & Schuster, 1993), 53.

21. Gerard Manley Hopkins, "God's Grandeur," in *A Hopkins Reader*, ed. John Pick (New York: Oxford University Press, 1953), 13.

22. Augustine, *Concerning the City of God against the Pagans*, trans. Henry Bettenson (London: Penguin, 2003), bk. 13, chap. 10 (pp. 518–19).

23. Arthur C. McGill, *Death and Life: An American Theology* (Eugene, OR: Wipf & Stock, 1987), 54.

Chapter 9: Just Community

1. Brad Gooch, *Flannery: A Life of Flannery O'Connor* (New York: Little, Brown, 2009), 365.

2. Kathleen Feeley, *Flannery O'Connor: Voice of the Peacock* (New Brunswick, NJ: Rutgers University Press, 1972), 11.

3. "Statement of the 1st Meeting of the IHR Emergency Committee on the 2014 Ebola Outbreak in West Africa," World Health Organization, August 8, 2014, accessed April 12, 2016, http://www.who.int/mediacentre/news/statements /2014/ebola-20140808/en/.

4. Andrew S. Boozary, Paul E. Farmer, and Ashish K. Jha, "The Ebola Outbreak, Fragile Health Systems, and Quality as a Cure," *Journal of the American Medical Association* 312 (2014): 1,859–60.

5. The three contiguous countries involved were Liberia, Sierra Leone, and Guinea. With nearly thirty thousand cases and over ten thousand deaths, it was a devastating epidemic for these relatively small countries.

6. Rudyard Kipling, "We and They," *Complete Verse* (New York: Doubleday, 1940), 768.

7. A famous section from the poetry of John Donne expresses the concept of shared vulnerability in evocative metaphor: "No man is an Iland, intire of it selfe; every man is a peece of the Continent, a part of the maine; if a clod bee washed away by the Sea, Europe is the lesse, as well as if a Promontorie were, as well as if a Mannor of thy friends, or if thine owne were; Any Mans death diminishes me, because I am involved in Mankinde; And therefore, never send to know for whom the bell tolls; It tolls for thee." See John Donne, Meditation XVII, *Devotions upon Emergent Occasions*, ed. Anthony Raspa (Montreal: McGill-Queen's University, 1975), 87.

8. See Matt. 14:13–21; 15:29–39; Mark 6:30–44; 8:1–9; Luke 9:10–17; John 6:1–13.

9. Wendell Berry, *What Are People For?* (San Francisco: North Point Press, 1990), 130–31.

10. Victor R. Fuchs, "More Variation in Use of Care, More Flat-Of-The-Curve Medicine," *Health Affairs* (2004 suppl): var104-var-107.

11. Eliot Fischer et al., *Health Care Spending, Quality, and Outcomes: More Isn't Always Better: A Dartmouth Atlas Project Topic Brief* (Trustees of Dartmouth College, 2009).

12. This number is changing since the Affordable Care Act of 2010. About five years after its inception, the rate of uninsurance has dropped to under 12 percent. Prior to this, the number of individuals without insurance was closer to 18 percent. See Ezekiel J. Emanuel, "How Well Is the Affordable Care Act Doing?," *Journal of the American Medical Association* 315 (2016): 1,331–32.

13. John Medaille, *Toward a Truly Free Market* (Wilmington, DE: ISI Books, 2010), 41.

14. Ibid., 42.

15. Wendell Berry, *Another Turn of the Crank* (Washington, DC: Counterpoint, 1995), 90.

16. Richard Wilkinson and Kate Pickett, *The Spirit Level* (New York: Bloomsbury Press 2009), 132.

17. Ana V. Diez Roux et al., "Neighborhood of Residence and Incidence of Coronary Heart Disease," *New England Journal of Medicine* 345 (2001): 99–106; Amy J Schulz et al., "Social and Physical Environments and Disparities in Risk for Cardiovascular Disease: The Healthy Environments Partnership Conceptual Model," *Environmental Health Perspectives* 113 (2005): 1,817–25.

18. Wilkinson and Pickett's country analysis shows this to be at around $10,000; that is, when national income per person falls below $10,000, as is the case in many poorer countries, health suffers as per person income falls (Wilkinson and Pickett, *Spirit Level*, 7). Other studies have focused on per capita health care spending. Below a certain level of health care spending, roughly $2,000 per capita, health suffers. Above this number, additional spending on health care results in minimal improvements in health outcomes. See J. Appleby and A. Harrison, *Spending on Healthcare: How Much Is Enough?* (London: King's Fund, 2006). For comparison, health care spending in the United States was over $9,000 per capita in 2013.

19. Wilkinson and Pickett show that it does not matter what politico-economic approach a country uses to reduce inequality. Whether by greater equality of market incomes before taxes and benefits or a redistribution of very unequal incomes through taxes and benefits, how a society becomes more equal is less important than whether or not it actually does so. Wilkinson and Pickett, *Spirit Level*, 176–77.

20. Ibid., 180–87.

21. The distribution of wealth in a society has a long history and many points of view. As previously mentioned, Wilkinson and Pickett, in *The Spirit Level*, address it more at a political level, though not dependent on one economic model. From a faith perspective, many have been influenced by the example and writing of John Perkins. In his discussion of the good that can be done when Christians get involved in community development, he makes "Redistribution" one of his three "R"s of Christian Community Development, along with "Relocation" and "Reconciliation" (*With Justice for All: A Strategy*

for Community Development [Grand Rapids, MI: Baker, 2011]). His recommendation, dependent on the link between a change of heart and a change in behavior, provides the most stable form of transformation because it is rooted in the deepest level of change. It connects to a story of biblical redistribution of profound proportions, when a wealthy tax collector named Zacchaeus meets Jesus in Luke 19 and through this life-changing experience, promises to "give half of my possessions to the poor, and if I have cheated anybody out of anything, I will pay back four times the amount" (Luke 19:8).

22. C. O'Donoghue et al., "Aggregate Cost of Mammography Screening in the United States: Comparison of Current Practice and Advocated Guidelines," *Annals of Internal Medicine* 160 (2014): 145–53.

23. Steven Woloshin and Lisa M. Schwartz, "The Benefits and Harms of Mammography Screening: Understanding the Trade-offs," *Journal of the American Medical Association* 303 (2010): 164–65.

24. See, e.g., Ex. 22:21; 23:9; Lev. 19:33; Deut. 10:17–19; 15:15; 24:17–22.

25. Among numerous references, see Isa. 1:15–17; 10:1; Jer. 5:27–28; 7:3–8; and Amos 2:6–7; 5:11–12.

26. For a beautiful description of the love and dedication of the Good Shepherd for his sheep, see John 10:1–18.

27. A pastor at a church hard at work for justice in a community in Washington, DC, once said in regard to our efforts, "What we do is important, but it doesn't really matter." At first I could not grasp the paradox, as I labored under the weight of the injustice around me as if it was all my burden to bear. Then I read Isaiah 42, regarding the chosen servant of the Lord: "I will put my Spirit on him, and he will bring justice to the nations. . . . In faithfulness he will bring forth justice; he will not falter or be discouraged till he establishes justice on earth" (vv. 1, 3, 4). For those that follow God's chosen servant, Jesus Christ, we know that the justice we work for is inevitable, because Jesus Christ will accomplish it. Karl Barth comes to a similar conclusion in the light of this eschatological perspective: "Hence we cannot allot final seriousness to what we do here and now. . . . We have simply to realize that we are children, and will be so to the very end, in whatever we do, because the perfect has still to come beyond all that we do now. . . . We cannot be more grimly in earnest about life than when we resign ourselves to the fact that we can only play." Karl Barth, *Ethics*, ed. Dietrich Braun, trans. Geoffrey W. Bromiley (New York: Seabury, 1981), 505. People who "play" purposefully can stay focused and stay at it for a very long time, even for a lifetime, making our work for justice a doable and durable effort.

28. Dietrich Bonhoeffer, *Ethics* (Minneapolis: Fortress Press, 2009), 161–62.

29. In Luke 16:19–31 Jesus tells the story of a rich man dressed in fine clothes and living in luxury who routinely passes by Lazarus, a beggar who is poor and sick. After death, Lazarus is carried to heaven and rests at Abraham's side, while the rich man ends up in hell, where he cries out for relief from his torment. But the separation between them is much too far for any help to cross. The reversal of fortunes and finality of destination that this parable portrays makes for a sobering reflection.

30. David Freeman Hawke, *Benjamin Rush: Revolutionary Gadfly* (Indianapolis: Bobbs-Merrill, 1971), 242.

31. Ibid., 243.

Chapter 10: The Cooperation of Faith and Medicine

1. David Cayley, *The Rivers North of the Future: The Testament of Ivan Illich* (Toronto: House of Anansi, 2005), 121.

2. For the remainder of this chapter, I will use the term *medicine* to refer to both the institution of medicine and the profession of medicine. Sometimes they are not the same, as when the practitioner of the art of medicine is trying to function at the highest level of his or her calling while the institution of medicine misuses its power as an impersonal system. At other times both the profession and the institution are corrupted by greed and a desire for prestige, or both are aligned for the good of the patient. In either case, both can be better for a healthier relationship with faith and religion.

3. Charles Taylor, *A Secular Age* (Cambridge, MA: Belknap Press, 2007), 270–88.

4. Lesslie Newbigin, *Foolishness to the Greeks: The Gospel and Western Culture* (Grand Rapids, MI: Eerdmans, 1986), 70.

5. Wendell Berry, *Life Is a Miracle: An Essay Against Modern Superstition* (Berkeley, CA: Counterpoint, 2000), 99.

6. Walter Percy, *Signposts in a Strange Land* (New York: Farrar, Strauss & Giroux, 1991), 297.

7. I started with the broad terms of faith and religion in discussing their assumed polarity with science. Now coming to specific problems and applications, however, the focus will be on what I know best: the Christian faith and the church. I leave it to the reader to widen the application to other faiths according to their own experience.

8. Jesus will later allude to this event and apply its symbolism to his own life, more specifically his death on a cross (see John 3:14; also 12:32).

9. The famous story of the Grand Inquisitor, told in Fyodor Dostoyevsky's book *The Brothers Karamazov*, demonstrates in sharp and uncomfortable lines our distaste for God's seeming ineffectiveness. Once again, Jesus is on trial, but now before the Grand Inquisitor in the 1500s during the time of the Spanish Inquisition. Unlike the Pharisees and Sadducees who condemned him to death the first time, this religious man is not threatened by Jesus's power. Rather, it is because Jesus has not used his power to solve the world's problems that the Grand Inquisitor finds him guilty and sentences him to be burned at the stake.

10. Henry Alford, *The Works of John Donne, Dean of St. Paul's, 1621–1631; With a Memoir of His Life*, vol. 6 (1839; repr. London: Forgotten, 2013), 244–45.

11. Quoted by Linda Treolar, "Reflections on Disability, Life, and God," in *Aging, Death, and the Quest for Immortality*, ed. C. Ben Mitchell, Robert D. Orr, and Susan A. Salladay (Grand Rapids, MI: Eerdmans, 2004), 166.

12. Traditional medical virtues guide the profession to put patient interest above self-interest and commit to caring for all patients independent of and prior to any consideration concerning their worth to society. Fidelity to these virtues allows patients to trust in the doctor-patient relationship. These foundations derive from the concept of a profession as a way of life in which the expert knowledge that the profession possesses is not for personal gain but for the

benefit of those who need that knowledge. The professions are in danger of forgetting these traditions, and the church is in a position to help them remember. For further reading on the ethics and virtues of the medical professional, see Edmund D. Pelligrino, "Character, Virtue, and Self-Interest in the Ethics of the Professions," *Journal of Contemporary Health Law and Policy* 5 (1989): 53–73.

13. Many others have offered much greater insight on the role of the church. For a thoughtful discussion of the sacraments and liturgy in relation to the body and medicine, see Joel Shuman and Brian Volck, *Reclaiming the Body: Christians and the Faithful Use of Modern Medicine* (Grand Rapids, MI: Brazos Press, 2006), 55–74. For a practical discussion of programs of health possible within congregations, see Mary Chase-Ziolek, *Health, Healing, and Wholeness: Engaging Congregations in Ministries of Health* (Cleveland: Pilgrim Press, 2005). For further thoughts on suffering, a few of the many resources include: Stanley Hauerwas, *God, Medicine and Suffering* (Grand Rapids, MI: Eerdmans, 1990); Stanley Hauerwas, *Suffering Presence* (Notre Dame, IN: University of Notre Dame Press, 1986), 23–87; Timothy Keller, *Walking with God through Pain and Suffering* (New York: Penguin, 2013); and Allen Verhey, *Reading the Bible in the Strange World of Medicine* (Grand Rapids, MI: Eerdmans, 2003), 99–145.

14. For further information on the role of the church in the uplift of disenfranchised communities, consult the Christian Community Development Association at http://www.ccda.org/.

15. For further information on faith-based health care for these communities, consult Christian Community Health Fellowship at https://www.cchf.org/.

Conclusion

1. While the Gospel writers acknowledge demonic influence in this setting, the word used for his condition suggests a more flexible view. In Matt. 4:24, a distinction is made between being demon possessed (*daimonizomai*) and having seizures (*selēniazomai*), suggesting less specific forces at work. In our passages, the boy's condition is *selēniazomai*, also translated as "moonstruck," which aligns with early beliefs that the frequency of seizures was related to the cycle of the moon. In either case, it is a destructive supernatural power that is causing illness and needs healing.

2. Edmund Fuller, *Man in Modern Fiction: Some Minority Opinions on Contemporary American Writing* (New York: Random House, 1958), 163–64.

3. Charles Taylor, *A Secular Age* (Cambridge, MA: Belknap Press, 2007), 547.

4. Allen Verhey, *Nature and Altering It* (Grand Rapids, MI: Eerdmans, 2010), 9.

5. Taylor, *Secular Age*, 548.

6. Josef Pieper, *Leisure: The Basis of Culture* (San Francisco: Ignatius Press, 2009), 116.

7. Ibid., 115.

8. Ibid., 116.

9. Ibid., 117.

10. Ibid.

11. Lewis Carroll, *Alice's Adventures in Wonderland and Through the Looking-Glass* (New York: Schocken, 1979), 167.

General Index

Scripture Index

THE GOSPEL **COALITION**

The Gospel Coalition is a fellowship of evangelical churches deeply committed to renewing our faith in the gospel of Christ and to reforming our ministry practices to conform fully to the Scriptures. We have committed ourselves to invigorating churches with new hope and compelling joy based on the promises received by grace alone through faith alone in Christ alone.

We desire to champion the gospel with clarity, compassion, courage, and joy—gladly linking hearts with fellow believers across denominational, ethnic, and class lines. We yearn to work with all who, in addition to embracing our confession and theological vision for ministry, seek the lordship of Christ over the whole of life with unabashed hope in the power of the Holy Spirit to transform individuals, communities, and cultures.

Join the cause and visit TGC.org for fresh resources that will equip you to love God with all your heart, soul, mind, and strength, and to love your neighbor as yourself.

TGC.org